WORK

AND

ALCOHOL ABUSE

Recent Titles in
Bibliographies and Indexes in Sociology

WORK

AND

ALCOHOL ABUSE

An Annotated Bibliography

Compiled by

John J. Miletich

Bibliographies and Indexes in Sociology, Number 12

GREENWOOD PRESS
New York• Westport, Connecticut • London

Library of Congress Cataloging-in-Publication Data

Miletich, John J.
  Work and alcohol abuse.

  (Bibliographies and indexes in sociology, ISSN
0742-6895 ; no. 12)
    Includes indexes.
    1. Alcoholism and employment—Bibliography. I. Title.
II. Series.
Z7164.C81M619 1987 [HF5549.5.A47] 016.33125 87-23619
ISBN 0-313-25689-6 (lib. bdg. : alk. paper)

British Library Cataloguing in Publication Data is available.

Library of Congress Catalog Card Number: 87-23619
ISBN: 0-313-25689-6
ISSN: 0742-6895

First published in 1987

Greenwood Press, Inc.
88 Post Road West, Westport, Connecticut 06881

Printed in the United States of America

The paper used in this book complies with the
Permanent Paper Standard issued by the National
Information Standards Organization (Z39.48-1984).

10 9 8 7 6 5 4 3 2 1

In memory

of

Dr. Peter Melling

Victoria, B.C.

Contents

Preface

A major difficulty in discussing alcohol use--and abuse--
involves semantics. Many words and expressions, and nuances,
are associated with the consumption of beer, wine, and liquor.
A few of these are: "normal drinker," "moderate drinker,"
"problem drinker," and "heavy drinker." Others include: "alcoholic," "substance abuse," and "alcoholism." "Drunkard,"
"inebriated," and "intoxicated" are three others. Many others, including slang expressions, could be added. Which words
most accurately describe something almost everyone can comment
on, either from personal experience or the experience of family, friends, or coworkers? It is not within the scope of this
preface to talk about this at length. The reader is referred
to the first chapter, "Definitions, Identification, Diagnosis."
An attempt will be made, however, to convey some idea of what
is meant by alcohol abuse, so the reader can have an initial
reference point.

     If one assumes there is a state of alcohol abuse, one can
ask: when does this state exist? Clearly, if people are nondrinkers, they do not consume beer, wine, or liquor, and there-
fore cannot abuse them. What about the drinkers who drink only
two cocktails daily, almost year-round? Do they abuse alcohol?
Perhaps. Perhaps not. This question could be answered easily
if there existed a precise, commonly accepted, universal definition of alcohol abuse. Currently, no such definition seems
to exist, for reasons such as the following. Although many
scientists and nonscientists believe that alcohol abuse is a
disease, there are critics of this disease concept. Alcohol
abuse is not a disease in the sense tuberculosis and yellow
fever are diseases; these diseases are definable more objectively than is alcohol abuse. Alcohol abuse can mean many different things to many people: a person either has or does not
have tuberculosis or yellow fever. Proving scientifically that
a person abuses alcohol is not as easy--perhaps it is not even
possible to prove scientifically--as proving that a person has
tuberculosis. There is, in 1987, much less stigma associated
with alcohol abuse, if the abuse is referred to as a disease,
than if the abuse is viewed as a character or moral problem.
This belief and relative lack of stigma, however, still do not

seem to properly categorize as a disease alcohol abuse along with yellow fever. There is a lack of specificity involved in defining alcohol abuse as disease, which is not involved in the definition of yellow fever.

Many variables--psychological, sociological, religious, philosophical, and physiological--enter into a clarification of the effects of "excessive" alcohol use on a drinker, and the effect of that drinker on those with whom he interacts. To the steadfast nondrinker, one drink, consumed by another person, can indicate alcohol abuse. Someone who opposes alcohol use, on religious or moral grounds, may maintain this view. Furthermore, abuse, whether in an alcohol or nonalcohol context, implies excess. But what is excessive to one person is not necessarily excessive to another. Four glasses of beer is excessive to someone accustomed to drinking one glass, but even four glasses are not excessive to someone who drinks eight. Some people, as is well known, "hold their liquor" well, meaning, in part, they have a better physiological tolerance to alcohol than do other individuals.

It is difficult, probably impossible, to state when "normal" or "regular" drinking becomes alcohol abuse. If one accepts the idea that no two people are alike in every respect, then no two individuals will become intoxicated in the same way, at the same time, by consuming the same amount of alcohol. One way of establishing a clearer picture of alcohol abuse is to think of a continuum. At one end are nondrinkers. At the other end are drinkers who died because of alcohol abuse. Somewhere between these two extremes are different starting points of alcohol abuse for different people.

Alcohol abuse, while not always apparent, is most apparent when the consumption of alcohol negatively affects people's lives. Relationships with family, friends, coworkers, and others are impeded, and quarrels, loss of friendships and jobs are attributable to excessive alcohol use. This provisional explanation is based on a review of literature for this bibliography and is not intended to be a definition. Even though one cannot provide a precise, commonly accepted, universal definition of alcohol abuse, one can state that the more people drink, the more likely it is they will become intoxicated. Over time--usually many years--they will probably die as a result of alcohol abuse. Cirrhosis of the liver is a typical cause of death, though pancreatitis and nutritional deficiency can also contribute to death. Most drinkers, if they do not become addicted to alcohol, and subsequently do not require increasing amounts, can lead productive lives for many years. Drinking, like smoking and eating, can become insidious over the long run. Drinking, it is true, does not "catch up" with every drinker. Every drinker does not die of alcohol abuse, just as every smoker does not die of lung cancer, and every compulsive eater dies not die of heart failure. But drinking too much, smoking too much, and eating too much inevitably

leads to ill health and death. It only takes a few years for
some people to reach this stage.

Alcohol abuse by employees is a major problem not only
for the employees themselves, but also for their employers,
coworkers, families, friends, and others. This is the situa-
tion worldwide in both government and the private sector.
Many employees who do not like their work drink before, during,
or after work to rebel against their jobs and supervisors.
Other employees drink because of marital, family, financial,
and other problems. For employers, this means decreased productivity, low employee morale, industrial accidents, absenteeism, and increased health care costs. The annual cost to
American industry alone is in the billions of dollars. The
cost worldwide is incalcuable.

Many companies located in the United States, as well as
companies in other countries, have found that it is more cost-
effective for them to rehabilitate employees who abuse alcohol
than it is to terminate them, and to hire new employees. Alcohol-abusing employees are informed that their work performance
is not at an acceptable level, that this is due to alcohol
abuse, that this abuse is a treatable illness, and that the employee, if he wishes to keep his job, will have to undergo
treatment at company expense. Rehabilitated employees are al-
lowed to return to their jobs. Those who refuse treatment, or
who cannot be rehabilitated, are eventually terminated. This
approach in dealing with alcohol-abusing employees has proven
to be very successful. Management and labor cooperate and most
employees are rehabilitated. Employee alcoholism programs--
the oldest in the United States date back to the early 1940s--
evolved into employee assistance programs. These latter programs offer assistance to employees, and even to family members, who have alcohol or other problems.

This English-language bibliography consists of over 1000
references, covering the fifteen-year period from 1972 through
1986. Source publications, all of which are annotated, include books, articles, dissertations, theses, conference proceedings, and government publications, most of which were published in the United States, Canada, and Britain. These and
many other countries are discussed in the seven chapters that
comprise the bibliography. References are arranged alphabeti-
cally by author surname. The chapters are: Chapter One,
"Definitions, Identification, Diagnosis"; Chapter Two, "Companies and Management"; Chapter Three, "Unions, Safety, Employee Dismissal"; Chapter Four, "Government"; Chapter Five,
"Specific Occupations"; Chapter Six, "Women"; and Chapter
Seven, "Counseling and Treatment." There are also separate
author, subject, and company-name indexes. The numbers in
these indexes refer to entries, not pages. There is also a
list of acronyms and a directory of sources.

This bibliography will be of interest to anyone concerned

about alcohol abuse in general, and about alcohol and the work-place in particular. Company and government employees at every level, including supervisory, middle management, and senior executive levels, can use this book as a sourcebook. Doctors, nurses, lawyers, and personnel staff are a few of the many professionals who will also find this book useful in their work. Sociologists, psychologists, economists, legislators, union executives, and social workers are others. Librarians at university, college, special, and public libraries can consult it daily in their work.

It is hoped the information in this book will help increase the knowledge of researchers and laymen, of a social problem whose costs--economic and human--are phenomenal.

I am very grateful to Mary R. Sive, Editor, Social and Behavioral Sciences, for her valuable guidance with this book--from initial idea to completed volume. Thanks also to Linda Grzywacz, Production Coordinator. I want to express my appreciation to the staff of the Alberta Alcoholism and Drug Abuse Commission Library in Edmonton for allowing me to use their excellent resources. Also, thanks to the interlibrary loan staff at the University of Alberta Library, who promptly provided me with information essential for the bibliography.

List of Acronyms

AA	Alcoholics Anonymous
AACP	Alcohol Abuse Control Program
AADAC	Alberta Alcoholism and Drug Abuse Commission
AAPPQ	Alcohol and Alcohol Problems Perception Questionnaire
AARR	Alcoholic At Risk Register
ABRL	Alcohol Behavior Research Laboratory
ADAMHA	Alcohol, Drug Abuse, and Mental Health Administration
ADD	Alcohol Dependence Data
ADS	Alcohol Dependence Scale
AFL-CIO	American Federation of Labor and Congress of Industrial Organizations
ALMACA	Association of Labor-Management Administrators and Consultants on Alcoholism
ALMEA	Alaska Labor and Management Affairs
ALPA	Air Line Pilots Association
AMA	American Medical Association
AMSA	American Medical Society on Alcoholism
APHA	American Pharmaceutical Association
APW	Alcoholism Program for Women
ARCH	Acceptance, Recognition, Confrontation, Hope

ARCO   Atlantic Richfield Company

ARF   Addiction Research Foundation

ARS   Alcohol Rehabilitation Service

ARTF   Alcoholism Residential Treatment Facility

ASI   Alcohol Stage Index

AT   Alcoholics Together

AUPE   Alberta Union of Provincial Employees

BAC   Blood Alcohol Concentration

BDI   Beck Depression Inventory

BFB   Behavior-Feeling-Behavior

BSCT   Behavioral Self-Control Training

CALM   Community Agency of Labor and Management

CAPC   Comprehensive Alcohol Planning Committee

CARE   Comprehensive Alcoholic Rehabilitative Environment

CBA   Cost-Benefit Analysis

CEO   Chief Executive Officer

CHAP   Corporate Headquarters Alcoholism Project

CLC   Canadian Labour Congress

CMD   Commission on Medical Discipline

CNR   Canadian National Railways

CNS   Central Nervous System

CP   Canadian Pacific

DANA   Drug and Alcohol Nurses Association

DOFASCO   Dominion Foundaries and Steel Corporation

DRLC   Drink-Related Locus of Control Scale

DS   Dogmatism Scale

DVR   Division of Vocational Rehabilitation

DWI   Driving While Intoxicated

EADS	Edinburgh Alcohol Dependence Scale
EAP	Employee Alcoholism Program
EAP	Employee Assistance Program
EHP	Employee Health Program
EMPOWER	Employee-Managed Program on Women Employees' Recovery
EPRA	Employment Program for Recovered Alcoholics
EV	Expected Value
FAA	Federal Aviation Administration
FRA	Federal Railroad Administration
GAO	General Accounting Office
GGT	Gamma Glutamyl Transpeptidase
GHQ	General Health Questionnaire
GM	General Motors
HDBQ	Hilton Drinking Behavior Questionnaire
HIMS	Human Intervention and Motivation Study
HS	Hopelessness Scale
ICL	Interpersonal Check List
IDAA	International Doctors in Alcoholics Anonymous
ILO	International Labour Organization
ITT	International Telephone and Telegraph
JCAH	Joint Commission on Accreditation of Hospitals
LAU	Leeds Addiction Unit
LEAC	London Employee Assistance Consortium
MAST	Michigan Alcoholism Screening Test
MCV	Mean Cell Volume
MCV	Mean Corpuscular Volume
MMDA	Multiphasic Matrix for the Diagnosis of Alcoholism
MMPI	Minnesota Multiphasic Personality Inventory

NABET   National Association of Broadcast Employees and Tech-
           nicians

NAIC   National Association of Insurance Commissiones

NASADAD   National Association of State Alcoholism and Drug Abuse
           Directors

NASAP   Navy Alcohol Safety Action Program

NBC   National Broadcasting Company

NBWA   National Beer Wholesalers Association

NCA   National Council on Alcoholism

NCAE   National Center for Alcohol Education

NIAAA   National Institute on Alcohol Abuse and Alcoholism

NMU   National Maritime Union

NNSA   National Nurses' Society on Alcoholism

NTSB   National Transportation Safety Board

NYSBA   New York State Bar Association

OAP   Occupational Alcoholism Program

OPAB   Ontario Problem Assessment Battery

OPC   Occupational Program Consultant

PAR   Program for Alcoholic Recovery

PMT   Power Motivation Training

QFV   Quantity Frequency Variability

QMH   Queen Mary Hospital

REAP   Railroad Employee Assistance Project

RSE   Rosenberg Self-Esteem Scale

SAAST   Self-Administered Alcoholism Screening Test

SADD   Short Alcohol Dependence Data

SADQ   Severity of Alcohol Dependence Questionnaire

SGOT   Serum Glutamic Oxaloacetic Transminase

SIT	Stress Inoculation Therapy
SPSS	Statistical Package for Social Sciences
STAQ	Spare Time Activities Questionnaire
TEAMS	Team Evaluation and Management System
TM	Transcendental Meditation
UAW	United Automobile Workers
UCB	United California Bank
UPIU	United Paperworkers International Union
USW	United Steel Workers
VA	Veterans Administration
WAIS	Wechsler Adult Intelligence Scale
WBAMC	William Beaumont Army Medical Center
WFS	Women for Sobriety
WHO	World Health Organization

WORK

AND

ALCOHOL ABUSE

1

Definitions, Identification, Diagnosis

1.001   "Alcoholism Ruled Disease in Pennsylvania." Labor-Man-
        agement Alcoholism Journal 8 (September-October 1978):
        76-80.

        Alcoholism was ruled a disease in 1978 in the Court of
        Common Pleas of Allegheny County, Pennsylvania. The
        court case was that of Donald A. Wagner versus Crucible,
        Inc.

1.002   Anderson, Peter, Anne Cremona and Paul Wallace. "What
        Are Safe Levels of Alcohol Consumption?" British Med-
        ical Journal 289 (December 15, 1984): 1657-1658.

        Reports on a survey of individuals engaged in alcohol
        research in Britain. These individuals were surveyed
        in order to gather information about safe levels of al-
        cohol consumption. No consensus was obtained on rea-
        sonable guidelines for safe drinking. Includes alcohol
        consumption limits recommended by the Royal College of
        Psychiatrists and the Health Education Council. 1 ta-
        ble. 4 references.

1.003   Apfeldorf, Max, Phyllis J. Hunley and David B. Thomas.
        "Two MMPI Approaches for Identifying Alcoholics: Eval-
        uation and Implications for Further Research." Inter-
        national Journal of the Addictions 20 (1985): 1361-
        1398.

        The Minnesota Multiphasic Personality Inventory (MMPI),
        and the MacAndrew Alcoholism Scale, are discussed in
        relation to a sample of 309 domiciliary patients. Au-
        thor biographical information. Abstract. 1 table. 6
        figures. 63 references.

1.004   "Are You an Alcoholic?" New York State Bar Journal 56
        (January 1984): 18

        Twenty questions to determine the extent of a person's
        drinking problem. The questions are used by Johns

Hopkins University Hospital in Baltimore, Maryland. 2 illustrations.

1.005   "Are You Drinking Too Much?" U.S. News and World Report 80 (January 12, 1976): 67.

Twelve questions prepared by Alcoholics Anonymous (AA) to use in evaluating a person's drinking habits.

1.006   Beauchamp, Dan. "Clearing Up the Myths." Toronto Board of Trade Journal 66 (June 1976): 51-55.

Discusses the variables which constitute the myth of alcoholism, and contends the myth prevents society's recognition of the seriousness of alcoholism. Author biographical information.

1.007   Beauchamp, Dan E. "Alcoholism as a Disease." in Beyond Alcoholism: Alcohol and Public Health Policy, by Dan E. Beauchamp, 6-8. Philadelphia, PA: Temple University Press, 1980.

Historical look at alcoholism as a disease. Makes reference to the views of physicians such as Thomas Trotter (England) and Benjamin Rush (U.S.).

1.008   Beauchamp, Dan E. "Constructing the Concept of Alcoholism." in Beyond Alcoholism: Alcohol and Public Health Policy, by Dan E. Beauchamp, 15-17. Philadelphia, PA: Temple University Press, 1980.

The focus of this section is on the work of Dr. Selden Bacon. Bacon was a sociologist who was Director, until 1976, of the Rutgers Center of Alcohol Studies, and a leading advocate of the disease concept of alcoholism.

1.009   Beauchamp, Dan E. "Is Alcoholism a Disease?" in Beyond Alcoholism: Alcohol and Public Health Policy, by Dan E. Beauchamp, 76-78. Philadelphia, PA: Temple University Press, 1980.

Comments on leading critics of the disease concept of alcoholism. Thomas Szasz, Claude Steiner, and David Robinson are three of these people.

1.010   Bell, R. Gordon. "Classification Systems of Alcoholism." in Classification and Symptomatology, by R. Gordon Bell, 9-19. Ottawa: National Planning Committee on Training of the Federal Provincial Working Group on Alcohol Problems, 1978.

After a look at the characteristics of classification systems, the Jellinek classification system is examined followed by a look at the Donwood Chart. Jellinek is

then correlated with Donwood. Major symptoms are explained and related factors in symptomatology, such as
nutrition, are elaborated on. This publication is part
of a series of publications on alcohol problems in Canada. 2 figures.

1.011   Bell, R. Gordon. "Popular Definitions of Alcoholism."
in Some Definitions and Parameters of Addictions, by R.
Gordon Bell, 9-11. Ottawa: National Planning Committee on Training of the Federal Provincial Working Group
on Alcohol Problems, 1978.

Among the definitions of alcoholism are the 1849 definition by the Swedish doctor, Magnus Huss, and the definition of Dr. E.M. Jellinek, in his 1960 book, The Disease Concept of Alcoholism. A 1971 World Health Organization (WHO) definition is also given. Some Definitions
and Parameters of Addictions is part of a series of publications on alcohol problems in Canada.

1.012   Bernadt, M.W., C. Taylor, J. Mumford, B. Smith and R.M.
Murray. "Comparison of Questionnaire and Laboratory
Tests in the Detection of Excessive Drinking and Alcohol-
ism." Lancet 1 (February 6, 1982): 325-328.

Approximately 400 adult psychiatric patients were investigated for this study. The patients were from two London hospitals--the Maudsley and the Bethlem. Eight laboratory tests were compared with three questionnaires.
The questionnaires were more effective in detecting excessive drinking and alcoholism. The Brief MAST (Michigan Alcoholism Screening Test), Cage, and Reich were
the questionnaires used. Author biographical information. Abstract. 4 tables. 32 references.

1.013   Bigus, Odis Eugene. "Becoming 'Alcoholic:' A Study of
Social Transformation." Dissertation Abstracts Interna-
tional 35: 3881A. Ph.D. dissertation, University of
California, San Francisco, 1974. Order No. DA7424460.

Analyzes the process by which individuals become alcoholics. There is a transition from normal social networks
to an alcoholic career. Normal social networks involve,
for example, family and occupation. Drinking behavior is
responsible for the alcoholic's eventual disengagement
from normal social networks. Interviews and participant
observation were used in this investigation.

1.014   Bissell, LeClair. "Diagnosis and Recognition." Chapter
in Alcoholism: A Practical Treatment Guide, edited by
Stanley E. Gitlow and Herbert S. Peyser, 23-45. New York,
NY: Grune and Stratton, Inc., 1980.

There are a number of things to look for in recognizing
and diagnosing the alcoholic. Noting how much a person

drinks is one of the things. Withdrawal symptoms, personality change, and blackouts are three other indicators. A physical examination which reveals secondary
diseases--cirrhosis and pancreatitis are two examples--
can also aid in identifying the alcoholic individual.
9 references.

1.015   Boscarino, Joseph. "Alcohol Career Patterns in Alcoholics Anonymous: A Systemic Approach to Alcoholic Defined Behavior." _Dissertation Abstracts International_
38: 6353A. Ph.D. dissertation, New York University,
1977. Order No. DA7803065.

This dissertation attempts, with the aid of a deviant
career concept, to explain alcoholic behavior, using
sociological and social psychology data. The deviant
career concept is used to explain how people come to be
affiliated with Alcoholics Anonymous (AA). This concept could enhance the understanding of deviant and
non-deviant behavioral phenomena.

1.016   Breitenbucher, Frances Joan. "The Concept of Alcohol-
ism." _Dissertation Abstracts International_ 42: 5052A.
Ph.D. dissertation, Georgia State University, 1982.
Order No. DA8212699.

What is alcoholism? What are its etiological determi-
nants? This dissertation examines these and other questions. There are over one hundred definitions of the
term "alcoholism."

1.017   Brisolara, Ashton. "Alcohol." Chapter in _The Alcoholic Employee: A Handbook of Useful Guidelines_, by Ashton Brisolara, 34-57. New York, NY: Human Sciences
Press, 1979.

Considers the question: why do people drink? Describes
what happens when a person drinks. Outlines twenty-five
signs of alcoholism. Lists twenty physical complica-
tions associated with alcoholism. Includes sixteen types
of treatment. 8 diagrams. 1 chart.

1.018   Bucky, Steven F. "Signs and Symptoms." Chapter in _The
Impact of Alcoholism_, by Steven F. Bucky _et al_, 1-10.
Center City, MN: Hazelden, 1978.

The four stages of alcoholism: pre-alcoholic stage,
prodromal stage, crucial stage, and chronic stage.
Gives eleven points to use in assessing alcohol problems.
1 table.

1.019   Caddy, Glenn R. "Alcohol Use and Abuse: Historical
Perspective and Present Trends." Chapter in _Medical and
Social Aspects of Alcohol Abuse_, edited by Boris Taba-
koff, Patricia B. Sutker and Carrie L. Randall, 1-30.

New York, NY: Plenum Press, 1983.

In addition to viewing alcohol use in historical perspective, recent trends in alcohol consumption, and alcohol consumption and alcohol problems, this chapter
also traces the development of the concept of alcoholism. This includes the traditional approach, social-
learning behavioral models, and the multivariate approach to understanding alcoholism. Advantages of the
multivariate approach are highlighted. 1 table. 130
references.

1.020   Caetano, Raul. "Diffusion of an Idea: Jellinek's Disease Concept in Latin America." International Journal
of the Addictions 20 (1985-1986): 1621-1633.

As the result of a visit to Chile in 1956 by Dr. E.M.
Jellinek, Chile and other Latin American countries--for
example, Argentina, Peru, Brazil, Costa Rica, and Mex-
ico--employ Jellinek's disease concept of alcoholism in
their studies of alcohol problems. Author biographical
information. Abstract. 1 table. 5 notes. 51 references.

1.021   Cahalan, Don and Robin Room. "Defining and Measuring
Drinking Problems." Chapter in Problem Drinking among
American Men, by Don Cahalan and Robin Room, 4-28. New
Brunswick, NJ: Rutgers Center of Alcohol Studies, 1974.

Many variables can be taken into consideration in defining and measuring drinking problems. Some of these
variables include: binge drinking, psychological dependence, belligerence after drinking, problems with
wife over drinking, problems with relatives, problems
with friends or neighbors, job problems, police problems over drinking, problems with health or injuries
related to drinking, and financial problems related to
drinking. 7 footnotes.

1.022   Cameron, Douglas. "How Abruptly Do People Get Drunk?"
in Aspects of Alcohol and Drug Dependence, edited by
J.S. Madden, Robin Walker and W.H. Kenyon, 66-70.
Kent: Pitman Medical Ltd., 1980.

Eight men, between the ages of eighteen and fifty-one,
were tested with a polygraph, in order to determine how
abruptly they became drunk. The subjects consumed or-
ange juice containing variable amounts of alcohol. A
breathalizer was used to measure blood alcohol concentration. The subjects reported the degree to which
they were drunk, since they were not told what constitutes drunkenness. Some stated they became drunk grad-
ually. Others said they became drunk quite abruptly.
This paper is based on the Proceedings of the Fourth
International Conference on Alcoholism and Drug Dependence, Liverpool, England.

1.023   Chick, Jonathan. "Alcohol Dependence: Methodological
        Issues in Its Measurement--Reliability of the Criteria."
        British Journal of Addiction 75 (1980): 175-186.

        This study was done in Edinburgh, Scotland and involved
        male patients at the Edinburgh Unit for Treatment of
        Alcoholism. The Edinburgh Alcohol Dependence Schedule
        was studied for its reliability to measure alcohol de-
        pendence. Author biographical information. Abstract.
        1 table. 21 references.

1.024   Chick, Jonathan. "Is There a Unidimensional Alcohol
        Dependence Syndrome?" British Journal of Addiction 75
        (1980): 265-280.

        Research could not demonstrate a unidimensional alcohol
        dependence syndrome. The research was done at the Roy-
        al Edinburgh Hospital in Scotland. One hundred and
        nine male subjects took part in the research. Author
        biographical information. Abstract. 5 tables. 19
        references.

1.025   Chick, Jonathan and John C. Duffy. "The Developmental
        Ordering of Symptoms in the Alcohol Dependence Syn-
        drome." in Aspects of Alcohol and Drug Dependence,
        edited by J.S. Madden, Robin Walker and W.H. Kenyon,
        54-59. Kent: Pitman Medical Ltd., 1980.

        Thirty-eight men were administered a structured inter-
        view concerning the developmental ordering of twenty-
        three symptoms in the alcohol dependence syndrome. The
        subjects, between the ages of twenty-one and sixty-five,
        were admitted to an alcoholism treatment unit. A se-
        quence was obtained resembling the classical description
        of alcoholism. This paper is based on the Proceedings
        of the Fourth International Conference on Alcoholism and
        Drug Dependence, Liverpool, England. 3 tables. 14 ref-
        erences.

1.026   Clark, William D. "The Medical Interview: Focus on Al-
        cohol Problems." Hospital Practice 20 (November 30,
        1985): 59, 62, 65 and 68.

        This article begins with a brief look at alcoholism as
        a disease then gives general strategies to aid clini-
        cians in interviewing potential alcoholics. This is
        followed by the physician's therapeutic role in treating
        alcoholic patients. Questions to ask during the inter-
        view are included. Author biographical information. 10
        references.

1.027   Clement, Sue. "The Identification of Alcohol-Related
        Problems by General Practitioners." British Journal of
        Addiction 81 (1986): 257-264.

In this British study, general practitioners, within the boundaries of Salford Health Authority, were sent a modified version of the Alcohol and Alcohol Problems Perception Questionnaire (AAPPQ). The purpose of the questionnaire was to measure the attitudes of general practitioners regarding patients with alcohol-related problems. The author learned that the attitudes of general practitioners are an extremely important variable associated with how these physicians identified and viewed alcohol-related problems. Author biographical information. Abstract. 4 tables. 1 figure. 17 references.

1.028   Cohen, Sidney. "Alcohol-Related Disorders: Early Identification." Chapter in The Alcoholism Problems: Selected Issues, by Sidney Cohen, 69-74. New York, NY: Haworth Press, Inc., 1983.

Alcoholic fatty liver, pancreatitis, gastritis, myopathy, blackouts, impotence, and cancer are some of the alcohol-related diseases or symptoms. 2 references.

1.029   Cohen, Sidney. "How to Become an Alcoholic." Chapter in The Alcoholism Problems: Selected Issues, by Sidney Cohen, 63-68. New York, NY: Haworth Press, Inc., 1983.

How alcohol consumption by an alcoholic differs from alcohol use by the person who does not have any problems with alcohol. A list of eleven indicators of alcoholism is included.

1.030   Cohen, Sidney. "The Many Causes of Alcoholism." Chapter in The Alcoholism Problems: Selected Issues, by Sidney Cohen, 85-90. New York, NY: Haworth Press, Inc., 1983.

The causes of alcoholism can be categorized into three main groups, with subgroups within each of the groups. They are: biological (for example, genetic or biochemical factors), psychological (learning theory or role modeling as explanations), and sociocultural (culture specific or subcultures under stress as the reasons). 4 references.

1.031   Cooney, Ned L., Roger E. Meyer, Richard F. Kaplan and Laurence H. Baker. "A Validation Study of Four Scales Measuring Severity of Alcohol Dependence." British Journal of Addiction 81 (1986): 223-229.

The four scales used in this study were: the Rand Dependence scale, the Severity of Alcohol Dependence Questionnaire (SADQ), the Last Month of Drinking Withdrawal scale, and the Last Six Months of Drinking Impaired Control and Dependence scale. Forty male and female patients, at the University of Connecticut, participated in the research. The subjects were interviewed

as well as asked to complete questionnaires. Author
biographical information. Abstract. 2 tables. 25 references. 1 appendix.

1.032   Criteria Committee National Council on Alcoholism.
"Criteria for the Diagnosis of Alcoholism." <u>Annals of
Internal Medicine</u> 77 (August 1972): 249-258.

Criteria for the diagnosis of alcoholism include physiological and clinical variables, and also behavioral,
psychological, and attitudinal factors. Abstract. 9
references. 2 appendices.

1.033   Davidson, Robin and Duncan Raistrick. "The Validity of
the Short Alcohol Dependence Data (SADD) Questionnaire:
A Short Self-Report Questionnaire for the Assessment of
Alcohol Dependence." <u>British Journal of Addiction</u> 81
(1986): 217-222.

Presents three studies which support the validity of the
Short Alcohol Dependence Data (SADD) questionnaire. The
SADD is compared to the Severity of Alcohol Dependence
Questionnaire (SADQ) and the Edinburgh Alcohol Depen-
dence Scale (EADS). Other research tools and tests used
were: the General Health Questionnaire (GHQ), the Drink-
Related Locus of Control Scale (DRLC), Gamma Glutamyl
Transpeptidase (GGT), and Serum Glutamic Oxaloacetic
Transaminase (SGOT). This research was done at the Leeds
Addiction Unit (LAU) in Britain. Author biographical in-
formation. Abstract. 3 figures. 3 tables. 23 refer-
ences.

1.034   Davies, D.L. "Defining Alcoholism." Chapter in <u>Alcohol-
ism in Perspective</u>, edited by Marcus Grant and Paul Gwinner, 42-51. London: Croom Helm Ltd., 1979.

Examines attempts to define alcoholism, including efforts by the World Health Organization (WHO). Also
talks about the disease concept of alcoholism and the
limitations of this concept. Questions the view that alcoholism is a form of drug addiction.

1.035   Davies, D.L. "Implications for Medical Practice of an
Acceptable Concept of Alcoholism." in <u>Alcoholism: A
Medical Profile, Proceedings of the First International
Medical Conference on Alcoholism, London, September 10-
14, 1973</u>, 13-22. London: B. Edsall and Co. Ltd., 1974.

Attempts to provide a simple, workable concept of alcoholism, one which does not view alcoholism strictly as a
disease. A discussion of this paper is included. 20
references. Abstracts in French and German.

1.036   Davies, D.L. "Is Alcoholism Really a Disease?" <u>Contem-
porary Drug Problems</u> 3 (1974): 197-212.

Alcoholism as a disease with reference to studies pertaining to Britain, the U.S., and Canada. Takes an ex-
tensive look at the disease concept of alcoholism as put
forward by E.M. Jellinek. Author biographical information. 1 figure. 20 notes.

1.037   Davis, C. Nelson. "Early Signs of Alcoholism." Journal of the American Medical Association 238 (July 11,
1977): 161-162.

Some of the early signs of alcoholism may include the
following: heartburn, morning cough, tachycardia, hy-
pertension, tremor in middle age, insomnia, hypergly-
cemia, and hepatic enlargement. Questions to ask when
there is a suspicion of alcohol abuse are listed.

1.038   Denenberg, Tia Schneider and R.V. Denenberg. "Alcohol
Abuse." in Alcohol and Drugs: Issues in the Workplace,
by Tia Schneider Denenberg and R.V. Denenberg, 159-160.
Washington, DC: Bureau of National Affairs, Inc., 1983.

Lists the symptoms of alcohol intoxication and alcohol
withdrawal.

1.039   Dittrich, Joan Elizabeth. "Alcoholism as a Diagnosis
among Clients and Their Spouses at Outpatient Psychotherapy Clinics." Dissertation Abstracts International
46: 3589B. Ph.D. dissertation, Memphis State University, 1985. Order No. DA8527048.

The Michigan Alcoholism Screening Test (MAST) was found
to be more reliable than psychotherapists in the diagnosis of outpatient alcoholics. Of patients whose spouses
drank, nearly 40% of the spouses were alcoholic, according to the MAST.

1.040   "Do You Have a Drinking Problem?" Toronto Board of
Trade Journal 66 (June 1976): 50.

Twelve questions to use as guidelines for evaluating a
person's drinking habits. Alcoholics Anonymous (AA)
prepared the questions.

1.041   Donovan, James M. "An Etiologic Model of Alcoholism."
American Journal of Psychiatry 143 (January 1986): 1-11.

A critical review of present-day etiologic models of alcoholism, and the introduction of a new model. The author first describes then critiques: trait studies,
psychoanalytic studies, hereditary/constitutional studies, sociocultural studies, and an interactional study.
After describing a new model of alcoholic etiology, he
talks about future research and implications for diagnosis and treatment. Author biographical information.
Abstract. 1 figure. 77 references.

1.042   Dreger, Ralph Mason. "Does Anyone Really Believe That
        Alcoholism Is a Disease?" American Psychologist 41
        (March 1986): 322.

        Alcoholism is not a disease, but rather a social phe-
        nomenon. Alcohol consumption is promoted not only by
        advertising, but also by peer pressure. A disease like
        tuberculosis is not promoted. Author biographical in-
        formation. 1 reference.

1.043   Dyer, Richard. "The Role of Stereotypes." in Images
        of Alcoholism, edited by Jim Cook and Mike Lewington,
        15-21. London: British Film Institute and the Maudsley
        Hospital, 1979.

        Stereotypes in general and particularly in relation to
        alcoholism. 16 notes.

1.044   Edwards, Griffith. "Case Identification and Screening."
        Chapter in The Treatment of Drinking Problems: A Guide
        for the Helping Professions, by Griffith Edwards, 177-
        182. London: Grant McIntyre Ltd., 1982.

        Why the diagnosis of alcoholism is frequently missed, en-
        hancing recognition rates, and laboratory tests and ques-
        tionnaire screening. 4 references.

1.045   Edwards, Griffith. "Causes of Excessive Drinking."
        Chapter in The Treatment of Drinking Problems: A Guide
        for the Helping Professions, by Griffith Edwards, 13-22.
        London: Grant McIntyre Ltd., 1982.

        A multiplicity of causes and not a single, isolated cause
        accounts for excessive drinking. Psychodynamic, environ-
        mental, and genetic influences are major causes. 21 ref-
        erences.

1.046   Edwards, Griffith and Milton M. Gross. "Alcohol Depen-
        dence: Provisional Description of a Clinical Syndrome."
        British Medical Journal 1 (May 1, 1976): 1058-1061.

        Among the essential elements of the alcohol dependence
        syndrome are: drink-seeking behavior, increased toler-
        ance to alcohol, repeated withdrawal symptoms, relief or
        avoidance of withdrawal symptoms by further drinking, and
        subjective awareness of compulsion to drink. Author bio-
        graphical information. 20 references.

1.047   Elkin, Michael. "Why Do People Get Drunk?: The Develop-
        ment of an Alcoholic System." Chapter in Families under
        the Influence: Changing Alcoholic Patterns, by Michael
        Elkin, 15-37. New York, NY: W.W. Norton and Co., Inc.,
        1984.

        The author believes people get drunk so they can become

powerful in interpersonal contexts. Drunks exhibit power-
er because they dictate the context in which behavior
occurs. Drunks with their drunkenness control other
people.

1.048 Estes, Nada. "Identification of Alcoholism." New Zealand Nursing Journal 76 (July 1983): 7-11 and 29.

The Cage Questionnaire and Short Michigan Alcoholism
Screening Test can be used to identify an alcoholic
person. Author biographical information. 1 illustration. 7 references.

1.049 Ewing, John A. "Detecting Alcoholism: The CAGE Questionnaire." Journal of the American Medical Association
252 (October 12, 1984): 1905-1907.

The CAGE Questionnaire consists of four questions and
was introduced in 1970. The questions, helpful in making a diagnosis of alcoholism, were developed in 1968 at
North Carolina Memorial Hospital. Author biographical
information. Abstract. 5 tables. 10 references.

1.050 Filstead, William J., Marshall J. Goby and Nelson J.
Bradley. "Critical Elements in the Diagnosis of Alcoholism: A National Survey of Physicians." Journal of
the American Medical Association 236 (December 13, 1976):
2767-2769.

Compares how the National Council on Alcoholism (NCA)
rates criteria for diagnosing alcoholism with the way
the American Medical Society on Alcoholism (AMSA) rates
the same criteria. Author biographical information. 3
tables. 12 references.

1.051 Fingarette, Herbert. "The Perils of Powell: In Search
of a Factual Foundation for the 'Disease Concept of Alcoholism'." in Drug Use and Social Policy: An AMS An-
thology, edited by Jackwell Susman, 568-589. New York,
NY: AMS Press, Inc., 1972.

Leroy Powell, the state of Texas, the disease concept of
alcoholism, and the U.S. Supreme Court. The case, Powell versus Texas, resulted because Powell was convicted,
under the Texas penal code, of public intoxication. The
validity of the disease concept of alcoholism, and the
degree to which it can be used as a legal defense, is
probed. 78 notes.

1.052 Finlay, Donald G. "Alcoholism: Illness or Problem in
Interaction?" Social Work 19 (July 1974): 398-405.

Questions the disease concept of alcoholism. Proposes
that alcoholism may be due to faulty interaction with
family and others. Author biographical information. 27

notes and references.

1.053   Follmann, Joseph F., Jr. "Alcoholism as an Illness."
        Chapter in Alcoholics and Business: Problems, Costs,
        Solutions, by Joseph F. Follmann, Jr., 26-51. New York,
        NY: AMACOM, 1976.

        Six areas are discussed: the problem of defining alco-
        holism, causes of alcoholism, the problem of diagnosis,
        the problem of identification, the effects of alcohol
        abuse, and prevention. 13 notes.

1.054   Freedberg, Edmund J. and Shawn E. Scherer. "The Ontar-
        io Problem Assessment Battery for Alcoholics." Psycho-
        logical Reports 40 (1977): 743-746.

        The Ontario Problem Assessment Battery, a self-report
        inventory, has been used successfully with employed al-
        coholics. This article is about the use of this re-
        search tool with 172 male alcoholics and sixty-eight
        spouses. The advantages of this battery are outlined.
        Author biographical information. Abstract. 6 foot-
        notes. 1 table. 4 references.

1.055   Fulton, Archibald. "Alcohol: How Much Is Too Much?"
        Nursing Mirror 160 (May 8, 1985): 32-33.

        Recognition and management of alcohol problems in Scot-
        land. The author, a nurse, presented a paper on this
        topic in April 1985 in Glasgow, Scotland at the Trauma
        '85 conference. Author biographical information. 2
        photographs. 5 references.

1.056   Gitlow, Stanley E. and Herbert S. Peyser. "Appendix B:
        Criteria for the Diagnosis of Alcoholism." in Alcohol-
        ism: A Practical Treatment Guide, edited by Stanley E.
        Gitlow and Herbert S. Peyser, 247-266. New York, NY:
        Grune and Stratton, Inc., 1980.

        National Council on Alcoholism (NCA) criteria for the
        diagnosis of alcoholism. These criteria include physio-
        logical, behavioral, psychological, and attitudinal fac-
        tors. 2 tables. 9 references.

1.057   Glassner, Barry and Bruce Berg. "How Jews Avoid Alcohol
        Problems." American Sociological Review 45 (August
        1980): 647-664.

        Suggests the following account for avoidance of alcohol
        problems by Jews: alcohol problems are perceived as
        non-Jewish, moderation practices from childhood, insula-
        tion by peers, and avoidance repertoire. Author bio-
        graphical information. Abstract. 10 footnotes. 73
        references.

1.058   Goodwin, Donald W. "Genetics of Alcoholism." in Psy-
        chiatric Factors in Drug Abuse, edited by Roy W. Pick-
        ens and Leonard L. Heston, 199-218. New York, NY:
        Grune and Stratton, Inc., 1979.

        Twin studies, adoption studies, and genetic marker
        studies have been used to study the genetics of alcohol-
        ism. That alcoholism is familial has been confirmed by
        the author's evidence. Familial, however, is not synon-
        ymous with hereditary and the exact cause of alcoholism
        is still not known. This paper was originally presented
        at a Conference on Psychiatric Factors in Drug Abuse,
        Minneapolis, Minnesota, March 4-6, 1979. 40 references.

1.059   Goodwin, Donald W. "The Symptoms." Chapter in Alcohol-
        ism: The Facts, by Donald W. Goodwin, 34-47. Oxford:
        Oxford University Press, 1981.

        Psychological, medical, and social problems as common
        indicators of alcoholism. Preoccupation with alcohol,
        guilt, and amnesia are three psychological indicators.
        Medical problems usually relate to the stomach, liver,
        and brain. Murder, employee absenteeism, and traffic ac-
        cidents are three social indicators of alcoholism.

1.060   Goodwin, Donald W. "What Is Alcoholism?" Chapter in
        Alcoholism: The Facts, by Donald W. Goodwin, 29-33.
        Oxford: Oxford University Press, 1981.

        Uses autobiographical comments to help define alcohol-
        ism.

1.061   Heather, Nick and Ian Robertson. "Introduction: Dis-
        ease Conceptions of Alcoholism." Chapter in Controlled
        Drinking, by Nick Heather and Ian Robertson, 1-20. Lon-
        don: Methuen and Co. Ltd., 1981.

        After a look at the historical context of alcoholism,
        this chapter examines the Alcoholics Anonymous (AA) mod-
        el, Jellinek's first and second disease concepts, then
        gives psychological explanations of alcoholism. The
        chapter concludes with a look at the alcohol dependence
        syndrome.

1.062   Hershon, Howard. "Alcoholism and the Concept of Dis-
        ease." British Journal of Addiction 69 (1974): 123-
        131.

        Alcoholism as a disease is analyzed as an assertion, a
        question, and an answer. Author biographical informa-
        tion. 34 references.

1.063   Hesselbrock, Michie, Thomas F. Babor, Victor Hessel-
        brock, Roger E. Meyer and Kathy Workman. "'Never Be-
        lieve an Alcoholic.'?: On the Validity of Self-Report

Measures of Alcohol Dependence and Related Constructs."
International Journal of the Addictions 18 (1983):   593-
609.

The sample consisted of 114 men and women--sixty-seven
men, forty-seven women--who voluntarily underwent treatment for alcoholism at the University of Connecticut in
Farmington, Connecticut.   The Last Month of Drinking
Questionnaire, the Last Six Months of Drinking Questionnaire, and the MacAndrew Scale were three of six assessment procedures utilized.   The authors learned from this
study that information obtained from the sample was highl
reliable and valid.   Author biographical information.   Ab
stract.   5 tables.   25 references.

1.064   Hill, Shirley Y.   "The Disease Concept of Alcoholism: A
Review."   *Drug and Alcohol Dependence* 16 (December 1985):
193-214.

Provides evidence pro and con that alcoholism is a disease and examines the implications of accepting the disease concept.   Some of the issues covered include more
specifically: defining alcoholism, defining disease,
disease as defined in medicine, symptoms of alcoholism,
signs of alcoholism, alcoholism as a syndrome, and alcoholism as a disease.   Author biographical information.
Abstract.   38 references.

1.065   Hilton, Margaret R. and V.G. Lokare.   "The Evaluation of
a Questionnaire Measuring Severity of Alcohol Dependence."   *British Journal of Psychiatry* 132 (1978):   42-
48.

An evaluation of the Hilton Drinking Behaviour Questionnaire (HDBQ).   Author biographical information.   Abstract
3 tables.   17 references.

1.066   Hodgson, Ray, Tim Stockwell, Howard Rankin and Griffith
Edwards.   "Alcohol Dependence: The Concept, Its Utility and Measurement."   *British Journal of Addiction* 73
(1978):   339-342.

Conclusions drawn from experimental data can be influ-
enced by assessments of the severity of alcohol dependence.   Author biographical information.   Abstract.   19
references.

1.067   Hodgson, Ray J.   "The Alcohol Dependence Syndrome: A
Step in the Wrong Direction?"   A Discussion of Stan
Shaw's Critique."   *British Journal of Addiction* 75
(1980):   255-263.

Comments on Stan Shaw's critique of the alcohol dependence syndrome proposed by G. Edwards and several other
people, including M.M. Gross, and R. Room.   Author

biographical information. Abstract. 31 references.

1.068   Holden, Constance. "The Neglected Disease in Medical
        Education. Science 229 (August 23, 1985): 741-742.

        Teaching students and clinicians about alcoholism--de-
        tection and treatment--at the Johns Hopkins Hospital
        and School of Medicine.

1.069   Horn, John L., Kenneth W. Wanberg and Gordon Adams.
        "Diagnosis of Alcoholism: Factors of Drinking, Back-
        ground and Current Conditions in Alcoholics." Quar-
        terly Journal of Studies on Alcohol 35 (1974): 147-
        175.

        Comments on: classical alcoholism, the sociopathic-
        gregarious drinking syndrome, drinking related to mar-
        ital problems, current personal maladjustment, anxiety-
        hypochondrical neurosis, and introversion-extraversion.
        Author biographical information. Abstract. 7 tables.
        12 footnotes. 29 references.

1.070   "How to Spot and Treat Alcoholism." Business Week
        (May 25, 1974): 127 and 130.

        Extensively quotes Dr. Morris E. Chafetz, Director, U.S.
        National Institute on Alcohol Abuse and Alcoholism
        (NIAAA). An inset section is entitled: "Are You an Al-
        coholic?" This section lists twenty questions which can
        be used in identifying alcoholics.

1.071   Howland, Richard W. and Joe W. Howland. "200 Years of
        Drinking in the United States: Evolution of the Dis-
        ease Concept." Chapter in Drinking: Alcohol in Amer-
        ican Society--Issues and Current Research, edited by
        John A. Ewing and Beatrice A. Rouse, 39-60. Chicago,
        IL: Nelson-Hall, Inc., 1978.

        Covers: the disease concept, definitions, alcoholism in
        America, temperance, prohibition, studies of alcoholism,
        Alcoholics Anonymous (AA), and remarks on alcoholism and
        the future. 46 chapter notes.

1.072   Hudolin, V. "Concepts of Alcoholism: Implications for
        Treatment and Rehabilitation." in Alcoholism: A Medi-
        cal Profile, Proceedings of the First International Med-
        ical Conference on Alcoholism, London, September 10-14,
        1973, 23-29. London: B. Edsall and Co. Ltd., 1974.

        The medical model of alcoholism and why a sociomedical
        model might be a more appropriate way of explaining al-
        coholism. The views of a number of individuals who com-
        mented on this paper are included at the end of the pa-
        per. Abstracts in French and German.

1.073   Ivens, Ruby E. "A Test of a Sociological Causal Model
        of Alcohol and Deviant Drinking Patterns." Disserta-
        tion Abstracts International 41: 4187A-4188A. Ph.D.
        dissertation, Western Michigan University, 1980. Or-
        der No. DA8106682.

        Socialization and social integration were studied as
        predictors of level of drinking, using data for the
        state of Michigan.

1.074   Izadi, Bijan Moghaddam. "Algorithms for Aiding the
        Clinician in Medical Diagnosis and Referral: An Appli-
        cation to Alcoholism." Dissertation Abstracts Interna-
        tional 39: 6089B. Ph.D. dissertation, State Universi-
        ty of New York at Buffalo, 1979. Order No. DA7913894.

        The self-report questionnaire, the treatment facility,
        and the clinician were some of the variables used in
        the development of an alcoholic referral mathematical
        model.

1.075   Jabbonsky, Larry. "Check Yourself and Enhance Your Im-
        age." Beverage World 104 (December 1985): 56.

        "Check Yourself" is a breath analyzer that tells bar
        and restaurant patrons whether or not they are intox-
        icated. William W. Wolfe, President, E.B.A.S., Inc.--
        Freeport, New York--comments on this machine. 2 photo-
        graphs.

1.076   Jacobson, George R. The Alcoholisms: Detection, As-
        sessment, and Diagnosis. New York, NY: Human Sciences
        Press, 1976.

        Thirteen of this book's fifteen chapters are about dif-
        ferent methods of detecting, assessing, and diagnosing
        alcoholism. Major methods are: the Alcadd Test, Bell
        Alcoholism Scale of Adjustment, Iowa Alcoholic Intake
        Schedule, MacAndrew Alcoholism Scale, Manson Evaluation,
        Michigan Alcoholism Screening Test (MAST), and the Mor-
        timers-Filkins Test. 195 notes. Glossary.

1.077   Johnson, H.R.M. "At What Blood Levels Does Alcohol
        Kill?" Medicine, Science and the Law 25, No. 2 (1985):
        127-130.

        Research data was obtained from the Department of Foren-
        sic Medicine, St. Thomas's Hospital Medical School.
        Data pertaining to the death of 115 individuals--they
        died between 1972 and 1983--was analyzed. There were
        eighty-four men and thirty-one women, between the ages
        of twenty-five and eighty-one. The general conclusion
        of this study was that death can result from alcohol
        poisoning having a postmortem blood level above 250 mg
        per 100 ml. This paper was originally presented at the

Tenth International Meeting, Association of Forensic
Sciences, Oxford, September 1984. Author biographical
information. Abstract. 2 figures. 11 references.

1.078   Kaplan, Howard B., Alex D. Pokorny, Tom Kanas and Gary
        Lively. "Screening Tests and Self-Identification in
        the Detection of Alcoholism." Journal of Health and
        Social Behavior 15 (March 1974): 51-56.

        Patients at the Veterans Administration Hospital in
        Houston, Texas were the subjects of research. The
        Michigan Alcoholism Screening Test (MAST) was adminis-
        tered to two groups of patients. One group were "self-
        identified" alcoholics. The other group were "non-self-
        identified" alcoholics. The purpose of this study was
        to determine if the MAST could be used to identify in-
        dividuals not openly identified as alcoholics. Author
        biographical information. Abstract. 2 tables. 7 ref-
        erences.

1.079   Keller, Mark. "The Disease Concept of Alcoholism Re-
        visited." Journal of Studies on Alcohol 37 (1976):
        1694-1717.

        After discussing alcoholism as a disease, this paper
        presents viewpoints critical of the disease concept.
        The paper concludes, however, that alcoholism is a dis-
        ease. The paper was presented at the Annual Meeting,
        Alcoholism and Drug Problems Association of North Amer-
        ica, New Orleans, Louisiana, September 13, 1976. Au-
        thor biographical information. Abstract. 11 foot-
        notes. 65 references.

1.080   Keller, Mark. "On Defining Alcoholism: With Comment
        on Some Other Relevant Words." Chapter in Alcohol,
        Science and Society Revisited, edited by Edith Lisan-
        sky Gomberg, Helene Raskin White and John A. Carpenter,
        119-133. Ann Arbor, MI: University of Michigan Press,
        1982.

        Historical look at attempts to define alcoholism and
        the problems encountered in attempting to arrive at an
        accurate, commonly accepted definition. Makes reference
        to efforts by the Cooperative Commission on Alcoholism
        and by the World Health Organization (WHO) to define al-
        coholism. Talks about the work of E.M. Jellinek. 17
        footnotes. 47 references.

1.081   Kjølstad, Th. "Alcoholism--An Illness." British Jour-
        nal of Addiction 69 (1974): 133-136.

        Alcoholism is not a disease in the usual sense of the
        concept of disease. The alcoholic, when he is sober, is
        not ill as he would be if he were afflicted with another
        disease. The alcoholic can be viewed as having bouts or

episodes of illness. 4 figures.

1.082   Kodman, Frank. "Bartenders' Impressions of the Person-
        ality Traits of the Excessive Social Drinker." Journal
        of Alcohol and Drug Education 29 (Winter 1984): 19-22.

        Sixty-one bartenders in three communities--Columbus,
        Ohio; Cincinnati, Ohio; and Lexington, Kentucky--were
        interviewed. The interviewers were enrolled in a social
        psychology class. Six major findings of the research
        are given. Author biographical information. Abstract.
        2 tables.

1.083   Lacoursiere, Roy B. "Screening for Alcohol Abuse."
        Journal of the American Medical Association 244 (October
        3, 1980): 1559-1560.

        Recommends easy methods of screening for alcoholism.
        These methods include asking questions and laboratory
        procedures. Author biographical information. 3 refer-
        ences.

1.084   Landeen, Robert H., Amy J. Aaron and Paul E. Breer. "A
        Multipurpose Self-Administered Drinking Problem Ques-
        tionnaire." in Currents in Alcoholism, Volume I, edited
        by Frank A. Seixas, 381-397. New York, NY: Grune and
        Stratton, Inc., 1977.

        Many demographic variables were analyzed in this study:
        marital status, sex, age, age began drinking, schooling
        completed, school grade average, employment status (em-
        ployed or unemployed), usual type of work done, and
        sources of income. This research was presented at the
        Seventh Annual Medical-Scientific Conference of the Na-
        tional Alcoholism Forum, Washington, D.C., May 6-8,
        1976. Author biographical information. 3 figures. 4
        tables. 15 references.

1.085   Landrau, Yolanda Cortes. "Nurses' Attitudes and Their
        Ability to Identify Alcoholism in a Patient Situation."
        Dissertation Abstracts International 46: 3006B. ED.D.
        dissertation, Columbia University Teachers College,
        1985. Order No. DA8525491.

        One hundred and seventy-three nurses, with experience in
        a medical-surgical nursing unit, were studied regarding
        their attitudes and their ability to identify alcoholism
        in a patient situation. The nurses completed the Prob-
        lem Identification Questionnaire and Marcus' Alcoholism
        Questionnaire. The researcher also asked the nurses to
        provide demographic data.

1.086   Lawson, Gary, James S. Peterson and Ann Lawson. "Etio-
        logical Theories of Alcoholism." Chapter in Alcoholism
        and the Family: A Guide to Treatment and Prevention, by

Gary Lawson, James S. Peterson and Ann Lawson, 3-15. Rockville, MD: Aspen Systems Corp., 1983.

Disease concept of alcoholism, physiological, psychological, and sociological theories of alcoholism. 26 references.

1.087   LeMasters, E.E.   "Taverns and Alcoholism." in <u>Blue-Collar Aristocrats: Life-Styles at a Working-Class Tavern</u>, by E.E. LeMasters, 161-164. Madison, WI: University of Wisconsin Press, 1975.

Remarks of tavern proprietors concerning alcoholism.

1.088   LeMasters, E.E.   "Who Is an Alcoholic?" in <u>Blue-Collar-Aristocrats: Life-Styles at a Working-Class Tavern</u>, by E.E. LeMasters, 157-161. Madison, WI: University of Wisconsin Press, 1975.

Drinking behavior of blue-collar patrons--at a tavern called "The Oasis"--is used to help define alcoholism.

1.089   Lender, Mark Edward.   "Jellinek's Typology of Alcoholism: Some Historical Antecedents." <u>Journal of Studies on Alcohol</u> 40 (1979): 361-375.

An earlier version of this paper was presented at the Twenty-Ninth Annual Meeting, Alcohol and Drug Problems Association of North America, Seattle, Washington, September 1978. Author biographical information. Abstract. 11 footnotes. 59 references.

1.090   Lerner, William D. and Harold J. Fallon.   "The Alcohol Withdrawal Syndrome." <u>New England Journal of Medicine</u> 313 (October 10, 1985): 951-952.

How to identify the alcohol withdrawal syndrome. Increasing blood pressure, increasing pulse rate, and tremor are a few of the early symptoms. Grand mal seizures, hallucinations, and delirium tremens may appear in some patients twenty-four hours later. The authors believe this syndrome, although readily identifiable, is often overlooked in the general hospital. Author biographical information. 10 references.

1.091   Lew, Don.   "Alcoholism as Disease." <u>Journal of the American Medical Association</u> 223 (February 12, 1973): 800.

Questions the validity of the disease concept of alcoholism.

1.092   Lewinson, Thea Stein.   "Handwriting Analysis in Diagnosis and Treatment of Alcoholism." <u>Perceptual and Motor Skills</u> 62 (February 1986): 265-266.

Compares, with the aid of two samples of handwriting, how the handwriting differs for the prealcoholic and postalcoholic person. Author biographical information. Abstract. 1 figure. 3 references.

1.093   Lieber, Charles S. "Medical Issues: The Disease of Alcoholism." Chapter in Alcohol, Science and Society Revisited, edited by Edith Lisansky Gomberg, Helene Raskin White and John A. Carpenter, 233-261. Ann Arbor, MI: University of Michigan Press, 1982.

Alcoholism used to be thought of as a social or behavioral problem. Presently, however, alcoholism is viewed as a disease, particularly since cirrhosis of the liver is associated with 75% of all deaths attributed to alcoholism. Examined here are: alcohol and diet in the pathogenesis of tissue damage, mechanisms of the toxicity of alcohol, and a public health strategy against alcoholism. 5 figures. 70 references.

1.094   Lisansky, Ephraim T. "Why Physicians Avoid Early Diagnosis of Alcoholism." New York State Journal of Medicine 75 (September 1975): 1788-1792.

An internist gives seventeen conscious and subconscious reasons why physicians are reluctant to make a diagnosis of alcoholism. This paper was presented at the Second Annual Meeting, American Medical Society on Alcoholism, Johns Hopkins University School of Medicine, Baltimore, Maryland, October 29-30, 1971. Author biographical information.

1.095   Lockhart, S.P., Y.H. Carter, A.M. Straffen, K.K. Pang, J. McLoughlin and J.H. Baron. "Detecting Alcohol Consumption as a Cause of Emergency General Medical Admissions." Journal of the Royal Society of Medicine 79 (March 1986): 132-136.

The subjects in this study were people admitted to a hospital in London. Hospital staff were interested in detecting alcohol-related medical problems. Questioning was found to be the most efficient way of detecting these problems. Questionnaire, biochemical, and haematological screening tests were less efficient. Author biographical information. Abstract. 5 tables. 1 figure. 16 references.

1.096   Lowery, Shearon A. "Soap and Booze in the Afternoon: An Analysis of the Portrayal of Alcohol Use in Daytime Serials." Journal of Studies on Alcohol 41 (1980): 829-838.

Fourteen soap operas were studied. Drinking is a regular occurrence in these programs. Three patterns of alcohol use were identified: social facilitation, crisis

management, and escape from reality. Soap operas do not
accurately portray all aspects of alcohol abuse as expe-
rienced in real, everyday life. Author biographical information. Abstract. 8 footnotes. 2 tables. 16 references.

1.097   Lumeng, Lawrence. "New Diagnostic Markers of Alcohol
        Abuse." Hepatology 6 (July-August 1986): 742-745.

        Questionnaires and laboratory tests should be used in
        conjunction with one another in the diagnosis of alcohol-
        ism. The Michigan Alcoholism Screening Test (MAST) and
        the Self-Administered Alcoholism Screening Test (SAAST)
        are two questionnaires mentioned. Serum acetate level
        and elevated blood acetate are markers of alcohol abuse.
        A drawback of using only questionnaires is that they re-
        quire the complete honesty of the individuals completing
        them. Alcoholics, typically, are hesitant to be totally
        frank about their alcohol consumption. The combined use
        of questionnaires and laboratory tests enhances objec-
        tivity. Author biographical information. 49 references.

1.098   MacFarlane, Stephen J. "Alcoholism Treated as Illness."
        Benefits Canada 4 (January-February 1980): 24.

        Perception of alcoholism as an illness and the treatment
        of this illness in a Canadian context. Author biograph-
        ical information.

1.099   Macharg, Suzanne Jane. "The Use of the Natal Chart in
        the Identification of Alcoholism and a Comparison of Its
        Diagnostic Efficacy with the MMPI." Dissertation Ab-
        stracts International 36: 7213A. Ph.D. dissertation,
        University of Southern California, 1975.

        The astrological natal chart and Minnesota Multiphasic
        Personality Inventory (MMPI) were used to identify alco-
        holics. Thirty male subjects--fifteen alcoholics and
        fifteen nonalcoholics--were the sample. One of the au-
        thor's major conclusions was that the natal chart, as
        interpreted by astrologers in this study, could not
        differentiate between alcoholics and nonalcoholics. The
        author recommended further research into the use of as-
        trology in psychological phenomena.

1.100   Madden, J.S. "On Defining Alcoholism." British Journal
        of Addiction 71 (1976): 145-148.

        The views of a number of people--including Aristotle,
        Karl Popper, and E.M. Jellinek--are incorporated into a
        discussion on defining alcoholism. There is also a cri-
        tique of the World Health Organization (WHO) definition
        of alcoholism. Author biographical information. Ab-
        stract. 18 references.

1.101   Marcinkowski, Tadeusz and Zygmunt Przybylski. "Evalua-
        tion of the Cause of Death in Cases of Acute Alcohol
        Poisoning." Forensic Science 4 (1974): 233-238.

        Data for this study was obtained from the Department of
        Forensic Medicine of the Medical Academy in Poznan, Po-
        land. The researchers were interested in cases of poi-
        soning with ethyl alcohol. Data covered the years 1959
        to 1968 and indicated an increase of frequency of lethal
        poisonings with ethyl alcohol. Author biographical in-
        formation. Abstract. 1 table. 7 references.

1.102   Mayfield, Demmie, Gail McLeod and Patricia Hall. "The
        CAGE Questionnaire: Validation of a New Alcoholism
        Screening Instrument." American Journal of Psychiatry
        131 (October 1974): 1121-1123.

        The CAGE questionnaire consists of four questions and is
        used in detecting alcoholism. This study evaluated the
        effectiveness of this questionnaire at the Veterans Ad-
        ministration Hospital, Durham, North Carolina. The CAGE
        questionnaire was compared to the Michigan Alcoholism
        Screening Test (MAST). Author biographical information.
        Abstract. 1 table. 5 references.

1.103   McCormick, Mary A. "Checking Patients for Alcoholism."
        RN 47 (February 1984): 52-53.

        A six-part checklist for assessing patients for physio-
        logical effects of alcohol abuse. The six parts cover
        the following systems: central nervous, gastrointesti-
        nal, hematologic, endocrine, genitourinary, and skin
        musculoskeletal. The checklist has sixty-five "suspi-
        cious signs," relating to alcoholism. Author biograph-
        ical information.

1.104   McKechnie, R.J. "The Question of Drunkenness: Who's
        Drunk or Whose Drunk?" in Aspects of Alcohol and Drug
        Dependence, edited by J.S. Madden, Robin Walker and W.H.
        Kenyon, 1-6. Kent: Pitman Medical Ltd., 1980.

        Friends, colleagues, and patients of the author provided
        input regarding the author's attempt to define drunken-
        ness. This paper is based on the Proceedings of the
        Fourth International Conference on Alcoholism and Drug
        Dependence, Liverpool, England. 14 references.

1.105   McKechnie, Ron J. "How Important Is Alcohol in 'Alcohol-
        ism'?" in Alcoholism and Drug Dependence: A Multidisci-
        plinary Approach, edited by J.S. Madden, Robin Walker and
        W.H. Kenyon, 123-138. New York NY: Plenum Press, 1977.

        A psychologist writes that there is more to alcoholism
        than alcohol--that in order to understand alcoholism,
        drinking behavior should be examined in a large context.

Social and cultural factors have to be studied. Explaining alcoholism in terms of laboratory animal studies is
not sufficient. This research was presented at the Third
International Conference on Alcoholism and Drug Dependence, Liverpool, England, April 4-9, 1976. 8 figures.
2 tables. 36 references.

1.106   Millard, Richard Woodworth. "Application of Selected
Measures for Detecting Neuropsychological Impairment
among Alcoholics." Dissertation Abstracts International
46: 2817B. Ph.D. dissertation, University of Hawaii,
1985.

The Stroop Color Word Test, Thurstone Word Fluency Test,
Progressive Figures Test, and Mirror Drawing Test were
administered to thirty alcoholic subjects and thirty
control subjects. These tests aid in identifying skills
lost by alcoholics. The Mirror Drawing Test was found
to be the most effective test of the four tests used.

1.107   Mooney, Al J., III. "Pharmacologic Basis of Symptoms."
Consultant 23 (May 1983): 171-174 and 177.

Different levels of blood alcohol concentration (BAC),
and their effect on the central nervous system (CNS),
are discussed as a pharmacologic basis of symptoms of
alcoholism. Abstract. 1 photograph. Author biographical information. 1 table. 1 figure. 4 references.

1.108   Moore, Robert A. "The Diagnosis of Alcoholism in a Psychiatric Hospital: A Trial of the Michigan Alcoholism
Screening Test (MAST)." American Journal of Psychiatry
128 (June 1972): 1565-1569.

This investigation was done at the Mesa Vista Hospital
in San Diego, California. The sample consisted of 400
adult psychiatric inpatients--270 women and 130 men.
The Hollingshead Two-Factor Index of Social Position was
a major research instrument used. The Michigan Alcoholism Screening Test (MAST) proved to be very effective in
distinguishing between alcoholic and nonalcoholic patients. Author biographical information. Abstract. 4
tables. 13 references.

1.109   Morse, R.M. "Alcoholism: How Do You Get It?" Chapter
in Fermented Food Beverges in Nutrition, edited by Clif-
ford F. Gastineau, William J. Darby and Thomas B. Turner,
359-369. New York, NY: Academic Press, Inc., 1979.

Begins with a discussion of the common concepts in etiology of alcoholism and concludes that virtually every person can become an alcoholic. 11 references.

1.110   Morse, Robert M. and Richard D. Hurt. "Screening for Alcoholism." Journal of the American Medical Association

242 (December 14, 1979): 2688-2690.

Screening for alcoholism by physicians can be done in a
number of ways. Asking questions, using screening
questionnaires, interviewing spouses, and relying on
physical and laboratory findings are some of the major
methods of determining if a person is an alcoholic.
Author biographical information. 15 references.

1.111 Morse, Robert M. and Wendell M. Swenson. "Spouse Response to a Self-Administered Alcoholism Screening
Test." Journal of Studies on Alcohol 36 (1975): 400-
405.

A table compares a self-administered alcoholism screening test and the percentage of respondents giving answers indicating alcoholism. Patients, spouses, and
counselors completed the test, an expanded version of
the Michigan Alcoholism Screening Test (MAST). Spouse
response was 90% accurate. Author biographical information. Abstract. 1 table. 9 references.

1.112 Murphree, Henry B. "Some Possible Origins of Alcoholism." Chapter in Alcohol and Alcohol Problems: New
Thinking and New Directions, edited by William J. Filstead, Jean J. Rossi and Mark Keller, 135-165. Cambridge, MA: Ballinger Publishing Co., 1976.

Three major areas are covered: the initiation of drinking, factors serving to maintain drinking, and factors
serving to terminate drinking. This chapter was originally a paper presented at the Lutheran General Hospital's Symposium on Alcoholism and Alcohol Problems,
Park Ridge, Illinois, Spring 1973. 146 references.

1.113 "Nine Symptoms of Alcoholism." American Bar Association Journal 70 (March 1984): 81.

Information about the nine symptoms of alcoholism was
provided by the Glenbeigh Adult Hospital in Rock Creek,
Ohio.

1.114 O'Brien, Lawrence J., Peter H. Rossi and Richard C.
Tessler. "How Much Is Too Much?: Measuring Popular
Conceptions of Drinking Problems." Journal of Studies
on Alcohol 43 (1982): 96-109.

College students rated 4560 vignettes, involving seven
independent variables, in order to judge the seriousness of drinking. Abstract. Author biographical information. 1 chart. 4 tables. 10 footnotes. 21 references.

1.115 Orcutt, James D. "Normative Definitions of Intoxicated
States: A Test of Several Sociological Theories."

Social Problems 25 (1978):   385-396.

Looks at intoxicated states brought about by marijuana
and alcohol. These states were rated positive or negative. The more individuals that used marijuana or alcohol, the less likely that the intoxicated state was
to be designated negative. The influence of friendship
is instrumental in defining an intoxicated state as
positive. The research sample for this study consisted
of approximately 1100 undergraduate students at Florida
State University. An earlier version of this paper was
presented at the 1976 Annual Meeting, Society for the
Study of Social Problems, New York. Author biographical information. Abstract. 3 tables. 4 footnotes.
28 references.

1.116   Orford, Jim. "Excessive Drinking." Chapter in Excessive Appetites: A Psychological View of Addictions, by
Jim Orford, 9-28. Chichester: John Wiley and Sons,
1985.

Historical and autobiographical information, from a
number of cultures, is used to examine excessive drinking. 1 figure. 3 tables.

1.117   Peele, Stanton. "The Dominance of the Disease Theory
in American Ideas about and Treatment of Alcoholism."
American Psychologist 41 (March 1986):   323-324.

The disease theory of alcoholism is discussed with reference to a number of studies and statistical data. 12
references.

1.118   Plant, Martin A. "Drinking Problems: Definition." in
Drinking Careers: Occupations, Drinking Habits, and
Drinking Problems, by Martin A. Plant, 11-12. London:
Tavistock Publications Ltd., 1979.

Gives definitions of alcoholism and common elements in
the definitions.

1.119   Pokorny, Alex D., Byron A. Miller and Howard B. Kaplan.
"The Brief MAST: A Shortened Version of the Michigan
Alcoholism Screening Test." American Journal of Psy-
chiatry 129 (September 1972):   342-345.

The authors found that the Brief Michigan Alcoholism
Screening Test--it consists of ten questions--was just
as effective in identifying alcoholics as the Michigan
Alcoholism Screening Test (MAST) which consists of
twenty-five questions. Author biographical information.
Abstract. 3 tables. 1 reference.

1.120   Popham, Robert E. and W. Schmidt. "The Biomedical Definition of Safe Alcohol Consumption: A Crucial Issue

for the Researcher and the Drinker." British Journal of
Addiction 73 (1978): 233-235.

Efforts to define a safe limit of alcohol consumption
have been attempted since at least 1870. More recent-
ly, such attempts have been made in Le Vesinet, France
at the National Institute of Health and Medical Research.
Since the average individual consumption of alcohol ap-
pears to be increasing throughout the Western World, research into defining a safe limit is justified. Author
biographical information. 14 references.

1.121   Preng, Kathryn Wallace. "Application of the MacAndrew
Alcoholism Scale to Alcoholics with Psychiatric Diagno-
ses." Dissertation Abstracts International 46: 1698B-
1699B. Ph.D. dissertation, Texas Tech University,
1984. Order No. DA8507458.

One hundred and forty male, veterans administration hospital patients were the subjects for this investigation.
These subjects were classified as representing one of
five groups: alcoholics, alcoholic personality disorders, alcoholic neurotics, personality disorders or neurotics. Each subject completed a MMPI (Minnesota Multiphasic Personality Inventory) from which MacAndrew Alcoholism Scale scores were determined.

1.122   Raistrick, Duncan, Geoff Dunbar and Robin Davidson. "Development of a Questionnaire to Measure Alcohol Dependence." British Journal of Addiction 78 (1983): 89-95.

Reports on the development of a questionnaire called Alcohol Dependence Data (ADD). ADD is a fifteen-item self-
completion questionnaire. It was administered to three
groups: regular drinkers, psychiatric patients, and alcoholics. Author biographical information. Abstract.
3 tables. 1 figure. 18 references.

1.123   Rankin, James G. "An Overview of Etiological Models and
Theories of Problem Drinking and Alcoholism." in Etiology by James G. Rankin, 10-14. Ottawa: National Planning Committee on Training of the Federal Provincial
Working Group on Alcohol Problems, 1978.

Moral, biological, psychological, and sociological models
of problem drinking and alcoholism are examined. This
publication is part of a series of publications on alcohol problems in Canada.

1.124   Ringer, C., H. Kufner, K. Antons and W. Feuerlein. "The
NCA Criteria for the Diagnosis of Alcoholism: An Empirical Evaluation Study." Journal of Studies on Alcohol
38 (1977): 1259-1273.

Two hundred subjects--120 alcoholics and eighty controls--

were studied, regarding the effectiveness of the National Council on Alcoholism (NCA) criteria for diagnosing alcoholism. The criteria were formulated in 1972 by an NCA committee. These criteria were very useful in identifying alcoholics in this study. However, the criteria were not without flaws. Approximately half of the controls were also diagnosed as alcoholics. Abstract. Author biographical information. 3 tables. 2 figures. 14 references.

1.125   Roebuck, Julian B. and Raymond G. Kessler. The Etiology of Alcoholism: Constitutional, Psychological and Sociological Approaches. Springfield, IL: Charles C. Thomas, Publisher, 1972.

Four chapters present definitions and incidence of alcoholism, as well as constitutional, psychological, and sociological viewpoints. 510 notes and references. 6 tables. 1 figure.

1.126   Royal College of Psychiatrists. "The Disease Model." in Alcohol and Alcoholism: The Report of a Special Committee of the Royal College of Psychiatrists, by Royal College of Psychiatrists, 54-55. London: Tavistock Publications Ltd., 1979.

Disease model of alcoholism.

1.127   Royce, James E. "The Disease Concept of Alcoholism." Chapter in Alcohol Problems and Alcoholism: A Comprehensive Survey, by James E. Royce, 159-176. New York, NY: Free Press, 1981.

Pros and cons of the disease concept of alcoholism. Prevention of alcoholism and the rehabilitation of alcoholics.

1.128   Rubington, Earl. "The Social Definition of Alcoholism." in Alcohol Problems and Social Control, by Earl Rubington, 68-69. Columbus, OH: Charles E. Merrill Publishing Co., 1973.

The social definition of alcoholism takes into account addictive (pure or habitue) alcoholics and symptomatic (essential or reactive) alcohoics.

1.129   Rudy, David Robert. "Becoming Alcoholic: Accounts of Alcoholics Anonymous Members." Dissertation Abstracts International 38: 5084A. Ph.D. dissertation, Syracuse Univeristy, 1977. Order No. DA7730756.

Data about Mideastern City Alcoholics Anonymous groups was used in this study. Participant observation and topical life history interviews were used to collect data. The author was interested in learning how an individual becomes an alcoholic, and was also interested in the process--series of events--by which that individual becomes a member of Alcoholics Anonymous (AA).

1.130   Saether, Claire D.   "The Alcoholic: Theory of Person-
        ality and Psychotherapy." Dissertation Abstracts Inter-
        national 46: 2078B. Ph.D. dissertation, Union for Ex-
        perimenting Colleges/University Without Walls and Union
        Graduate School, 1985. Order No. DA8518383.

        This dissertation views alcoholism as a developmental
        personality disorder--an alcoholic ideology. Treatment
        for alcoholism entails an ideological change on the part
        of the alcoholic.

1.131   Sanchez-Craig, Martha. "How Much Is Too Much?: Esti-
        mates of Hazardous Drinking Based on Clients' Self-Re-
        ports." British Journal of Addiction 81 (1986): 251-
        256.

        The gamma glutamyl transpeptidase (GGT), a liver func-
        tion test, was used to corroborate self-reported drink-
        ing. The Alcohol Dependence Scale (ADS) and the Mich-
        igan Alcoholism Screening Test (MAST) were also used in
        this research. The author was interested in the quan-
        tity and frequency of alcohol consumed by clients dis-
        charged from alcoholism treatment. Author biographical
        information. Abstract. 3 tables. 19 references.

1.132   Scaturo, Douglas Jerome. "Adaptation to Ethanol Intox-
        ication as a Potential Measure of Alcohol Abuse." Dis-
        sertation Abstracts International 39: 6141B. Ph.D.
        dissertation, Claremont Graduate School, 1978. Order
        No. DA7911546.

        Research involved male subjects who took part in three
        experiments concerning alcohol and the measurement of
        alcohol abuse.

1.133   Schlaadt, Richard G. and Peter T. Shannon. "What Is Al-
        coholism?" in Drugs of Choice: Current Perspectives on
        Drug Use, by Richard G. Schlaadt and Peter T. Shannon,
        Second Edition, 160-165. Englewood Cliffs, NJ: Pren-
        tice-Hall, 1986.

        Lists from the disease perspective six stages in alco-
        holism: the well individual, the episodic-excessive
        drinker, the habitual-excessive drinker, alcohol addic-
        tion--physiological changes, alcohol addiction--irrevers-
        ible damage, and death. Includes twenty-five specific
        cognitive-behavioral indicators by which alcoholism can
        be diagnosed.

1.134   Schuckit, Marc A. "Definition of Alcoholism." in Drug
        and Alcohol Abuse: A Clinical Guide to Diagnosis and
        Treatment, by Marc A. Schuckit, 38-39. New York, NY:

Plenum Medical Book Co., 1979.

Four variables can be taken into account in defining alcoholism. They are: the quantity-frequency-variability
(QFV) variable, psychological dependence, withdrawal or
abstinence symptoms, and social or health problems related to alcohol. Furthermore, there is no single,
best, overall definition of alcoholism.

1.135   Schuckit, Marc A. "Identification of the Alcoholic."
        in Drug and Alcohol Abuse: A Clinical Guide to Diagno-
        sis and Treatment, by Marc A. Schuckit, 53-54. New
        York, NY: Plenum Medical Book Co., 1979.

        Insomnia, nervousness, high blood pressure, and elevated
        uric acid can be indicators of alcoholism. Sadness, in-
        terpersonal problems, and ulcer disease can also be in-
        dicators.

1.136   Shaw, Stan. "A Critique of the Concept of the Alcohol
        Dependence Syndrome." British Journal of Addiction 74
        (1979): 339-348.

        The International Classification of Diseases no longer
        includes the term "alcoholism." This term has been re-
        placed by the concept of the "alcohol dependence syn-
        drome." Rationale justifying the syndrome idea is ex-
        amined. Author biographical information. Abstract.
        16 references.

1.137   Shaw, Stan, Alan Cartwright, Terry Spratley and Judith
        Harwin. "Concepts of Alcohol Abuse." Chapter in Re-
        sponding to Drinking Problems, by Stan Shaw, Alan Cart-
        wright, Terry Spratley and Judith Harwin, 41-76. Bal-
        timore, MD: University Park Press, 1978.

        Some of the topics: the history of concepts of alcohol
        abuse, Alcoholics Anonymous (AA) and the disease concept
        of alcoholism, criticism of the disease concept, alco-
        holism as a stigmatized illness, and the scientific ev-
        idence of dependence.

1.138   Sherin, Kevin. "Screening for Alcoholism." American
        Family Physician 26 (July 1982): 179-181.

        Three clues to alcoholism are heartburn, morning gas-
        tritis, and diarrhea. Financial and emotional problems
        are two social consequences of alcoholism. Liver dis-
        ease, elevated blood pressure, and tremors are physical
        and laboratory indicators of this disease. The Michi-
        gan Alcoholism Screening Test (MAST) can aid in the
        early diagnosis of alcoholism. Author biographical in-
        formation. 5 references.

1.139   Skinner, Harvey A. "Primary Syndromes of Alcohol Abuse:

Their Measurement and Correlates." British Journal of
Addiction 76 (1981): 63-76.

Alcohol dependence, perceived benefits from drinking,
marital discord, and polydrug abuse were identified as
major syndromes of alcohol abuse, when the Alcohol Use
Inventory was administered to a sample of 274 individuals. The individuals had sought help at the Clinical
Institute of the Addiction Research Foundation in Toronto, Ontario. Author biographical information. Abstract. 4 tables. 33 references.

1.140   Skinner, Harvey A. and Barbara A. Allen. "Alcohol Dependence Syndrome: Measurement and Validation." Journal of Abnormal Psychology 91 (1982): 199-209.

People who sought assistance for alcohol problems at
the Addiction Research Foundation in Toronto constituted the sample for this study. Of the 225 people who
participated, 80% were male, 20% were female. The average age was thirty-eight years. Research tools included: the Michigan Alcoholism Screening Test (MAST),
the Alcohol Use Inventory, the Lifetime Drinking History Structured Interview, the Wechsler Adult Intelli-
gence Scale (WAIS), the Basic Personality Inventory, and
the Cornell Medical Index. The purpose of this study
was to measure and validate the alcohol dependence syndrome proposed in 1976 by Edwards and Gross. Author
biographical information. Abstract. 5 tables. 4 figures. 42 references.

1.141   Skinner, Harvey A. and John L. Horn. Alcohol Dependence
Scale (ADS) User's Guide. Toronto: Addiction Research
Foundation, 1984.

This manual reviews published developments about alcohol dependence, describes the reliability and validity
of the alcohol dependence scale, and provides instruc-
tions for administering, scoring, and interpreting the
ADS. 6 figures. 9 tables. 47 references.

1.142   Skinner, Thelma Jean and K.D. Charalampous. "Interpre-
tive Procedures Entailed in Using the Michigan Alcoholism Screening Test." British Journal of Addiction 73
(1978): 117-121.

A study done at the offices of the Texas Alcohol Safety Action Project. The sample consisted of thirty individuals convicted of driving while intoxicated (DWI).
Results are reported in terms of: self-administered
MAST (Michigan Alcoholism Screening Test) versus counselor-administered MAST, counselor-administered MAST
versus counselor's diagnosis, and self-administered
MAST versus counselor's diagnosis. Author biographical
information. Abstract. 9 references.

1.143   Smith, James W.   "Diagnosing Alcoholism."   Hospital and
        Community Psychiatry 34 (November 1983):   1017-1021.

        Alcoholism, like syphilis, imitates other diseases.   In
        diagnosing alcoholism, it is important to consider ste-
        reotypes and definitions.   It is also important to dif-
        ferentiate between primary and secondary alcoholism.
        The orthopedic, cardiovascular, gastrointestinal, neu-
        rologic, and genitourinary systems, as well as the skin,
        should be examined when making a diagnosis.   Author bio-
        graphical information.   Abstract.   23 references.

1.144   Starr, Douglas.   "High-Tech Drunk Test."   Omni 8 (June
        1986):   41.

        Veritas 100 is a device which measures brain waves in
        order to detect the presence of alcohol and drugs in a
        person's body.   This device is more effective than, for
        example, a breathalyzer.   S. Thomas Westerman, a New
        Jersey ear, nose, and throat specialist, invented
        Veritas 100.   1 photograph.

1.145   Stockwell, Tim, Ray Hodgson, Griffith Edwards, Colin
        Taylor and Howard Rankin.   "The Development of a Ques-
        tionnaire to Measure Severity of Alcohol Dependence."
        British Journal of Addiction 74 (1979):   79-87.

        By 1978, there were approximately 360 questionnaires used
        in studying drinking behavior.   In this study, problem
        drinkers who were patients at the Maudsley Hospital and
        the Bethlem Royal Hospital in England were administered
        the Severity of Alcohol Dependence Questionnaire (SADQ).
        This questionnaire was found to be a valid instrument for
        measuring alcohol dependence.   Author biographical infor-
        mation.   3 tables.   12 references.   1 appendix.

1.146   Swenson, Wendell M. and Robert M. Morse.   "The Use of a
        Self-Administered Alcoholism Screening Test (SAAST) in a
        Medical Center."   Mayo Clinic Proceedings 50 (April 1975):
        204-208.

        A self-administered alcoholism screening questionnaire
        was given to 200 patients.   Half of the patients were be-
        ing treated for alcoholism.   The other half of the pa-
        tients were a random group in a medical population.   The
        questionnaire was successful in identifying the "hidden
        alcoholic" in the medical population.   Two case histories
        are included.   Author biographical information.   Abstract.
        1 table.   9 references.   1 appendix.

1.147   Tarter, Ralph E.   "The Causes of Alcoholism: A Biopsy-
        chological Analysis."   Chapter in Etiologic Aspects of
        Alcohol and Drug Abuse, edited by Edward Gottheil, Keith
        A. Druley, Thomas E. Skoloda and Howard M. Waxman,

173-201.   Springfield, IL: Charles C. Thomas, Publisher, 1983.

After a look at models of alcoholism, this chapter discusses differences between alcoholics and social drinkers. This is followed by genetic, biochemical, and psychophysiological theories regarding the etiology of alcoholism. A biosocial research program about the early age onset, severe drinker is discussed next. The chapter ends with an attempt at an empirical integration. This chapter was presented as a paper at the Fourth Jefferson Conference on Addiction, Coatesville, Virginia, 1980. 9 tables. 63 references.

1.148   Terbell, Thomas G.   "What's So Bad About Being an Alcoholic?" Labor-Management Alcoholism Journal 8 (July-August 1978):   22-23.

Comments on euphemisms for "alcoholism" and "alcoholics," and examines the implications for alcoholics, their employers, and other people. Author biographical information. 1 photograph.

1.149   Trice, Harrison M. and Paul M. Roman.   "American Drinking Norms." in Spirits and Demons at Work: Alcohol and Other Drugs on the Job, by Harrison M. Trice and Paul M. Roman, Second Edition, 18-21. Ithaca, NY: New York State School of Industrial and Labor Relations Cornell University, 1978.

Historical and sociological factors are used to explain American drinking norms. The Women's Christian Temperance Union and the Prohibionist Party are mentioned.

1.150   Trice, Harrison M. and Paul M. Roman.   "The Causes of Deviant Drinking and Alcohol Addiction." in Spirits and Demons at Work: Alcohol and Other Drugs on the Job, by Harrison M. Trice and Paul M. Roman, Second Edition, 25-28. Ithaca, NY: New York State School of Industrial and Labor Relations Cornell University, 1978.

The authors contend that the causes of deviant drinking and alcohol addiction have not been discovered. The validity of the disease model of alcoholism has been questioned. No widespread, accepted definition of normal drinking exists.

1.151   Trice, Harrison M. and Paul M. Roman.   "The Definition of Alcohol Problems." in Spirits and Demons at Work: Alcohol and Other Drugs on the Job, by Harrison M. Trice and Paul M. Roman, Second Edition, 12-18. Ithaca, NY: New York State School of Industrial and Labor Relations Cornell University, 1978.

A definition of alcohol problems entails historical

accounts of alcohol use, the disease model of alcoholism,
normal and deviant drinking, and alcohol addiction.

1.152   Trice, Harrison M. and Paul M. Roman. "Vulnerability
        Factors." in Spirits and Demons at Work: Alcohol and
        Other Drugs on the Job, by Harrison M. Trice and Paul M.
        Roman, Second Edition, 28-31. Ithaca, NY: New York
        State School of Industrial and Labor Relations Cornell
        University, 1978.

        Certain people appear to be more likely than others to
        become alcohol dependent. People who have problems of
        self-image, those who need to relieve anxiety and de-
        pression, and those who have a deviant drinker in their
        family may become alcohol dependent.

1.153   Twerski, Abraham J. "Alcoholism Defined." Chapter in
        Caution: 'Kindness' Can Be Dangerous to the Alcoholic,
        by Abraham J. Twerski, 8-18. Englewood Cliffs, NJ:
        Prentice-Hall, 1981.

        A medical case history and letter from an alcoholic to
        his doctor help define alcoholism.

1.154   Vaillant, George E. "Is Alcoholism a Unitary Disorder?"
        Chapter in The Natural History of Alcoholism, by George
        E. Vaillant, 15-44. Cambridge, MA: Harvard University
        Press, 1983.

        A look at the medical model of alcoholism. States that
        alcoholism should be viewed as both a disease and a be-
        havior disorder. Claims that psychologists are often
        more successful in treating alcoholism than are doctors.
        9 tables. 1 figure.

1.155   Wanberg, Kenneth W. and John L. Horn. "Alcoholism Syn-
        dromes Related to Sociological Classifications." Inter-
        national Journal of the Addictions 8 (1973): 99-120.

        According to this study, alcoholism does not appear to
        be a single syndrome, but rather a multidimensional phe-
        nomenon. Approximately 1900 male and female, alcoholic
        subjects constituted the sample. The research took
        place at the Fort Logan Mental Health Center, where the
        men and women were patients at the Alcoholism Division.
        Variables studied were: male and female differences,
        education, annual income, employment, ethnic groups,
        age, and marital status. Other variables investigated:
        gregarious-beer drinking versus solitary drinking, sus-
        tained versus periodic drinking, weekend and daily con-
        trolled drinking, psychological and social benefits,
        shame, resentment, and fear associated with drinking,
        and prior-help associated with drinking. Author bio-
        graphical information. 4 tables. 21 references.

1.156   Wanberg, Kenneth W., John L. Horn and F. Mark Foster.
        "A Differential Assessment Model for Alcoholism: The
        Scales of the Alcohol Use Inventory." Journal of
        Studies on Alcohol 38 (1977): 512-543.

        Three main areas: the problems with alcoholism theo-
        ries, the development of a differential model, and the
        benefits of the differential assessment model. Ab-
        stract. Author biographical information. 13 foot-
        notes. 1 chart. 2 figures. 8 tables. 32 references.

1.157   Watts, Thomas D. "The Uneasy Triumph of a Concept:
        The 'Disease' Conception of Alcoholism." Journal of
        Drug Issues 11 (1981): 451-460.

        Acknowledges the widespread acceptance of the disease
        concept of alcoholism--the concept's growth, develop-
        ment, and influence. Also talks about six areas, in
        particular, in which this concept's validity has been
        questioned. Abstract. Author biographical informa-
        tion. 36 references.

1.158   Weinberger, Martha Bernatz. "The Classification of Al-
        coholics: A Comparison of Two MMPI-Based Typologies."
        Dissertation Abstracts International 47: 1324B. Ph.D.
        dissertation, University of Alabama, 1985.

        One thousand male alcoholics were the sample for this
        research. These individuals were administered the Min-
        nesota Multiphasic Personality Inventory (MMPI). So-
        cial history, drinking history, and mental status were
        investigated.

1.159   White, Helene Raskin. "Sociological Theories of the
        Etiology of Alcoholism." Chapter in Alcohol, Science
        and Society Revisited, edited by Edith Lisansky Gom-
        berg, Helene Raskin White and John A. Carpenter, 205-
        232. Ann Arbor, MI: University of Michigan Press,
        1982.

        Six sociological theories are related to the etiology
        of alcoholism: sociodemographic, sociocultural, so-
        cialization, social deviance, socioenvironmental, and
        interactive. 13 footnotes. 51 references.

1.160   Wilkins, Rodney H. "The Detection of Alcoholism by a
        Non-Specialist." in Alcoholism: A Medical Profile,
        Proceedings of the First International Medical Confer-
        ence on Alcoholism, London, September 10-14, 1973, 186-
        194. London: B. Edsall and Co. Ltd., 1974.

        Patients at the Manchester University Department of
        General Practice were asked to complete questionnaires,
        in order to determine to what extent each patient abused
        alcohol. The two questionnaires used were the Alcoholic

At Risk Register (AARR) and the Spare Time Activities
Questionnaire (STAQ). The text of a discussion of this
paper is included. 26 references. Abstracts in French
and German.

1.161   Wilkinson, A. Earl. "The Alcohol Abuser." Chapter in
        Types of Drug Abusers and Their Abuses, by John G. Cull
        and Richard E. Hardy, 146-159. Springfield, IL: Charles
        C. Thomas, Publisher, 1974.

        Four topics are covered: physiological and psychologi-
        cal effects of alcohol ingestion, patterns and phases
        of alcohol abuse, causes of alcoholism, and treatment of
        the alcohol abuser. 30 references.

1.162   Willoughby, Alan. "A Good Working Definition." Chapter
        in The Alcohol Troubled Person: Known and Unknown, by
        Alan Willoughby, 65-125. Chicago, IL: Nelson-Hall,
        Inc., 1979.

        Social, financial, physical, and emotional components
        are used in a working definition of alcoholism. Also
        associated with alcoholism are: avitaminosis, cirrho-
        sis of the liver, peripheral neuropathy, gastritis and
        ulcers, diabetes, tuberculosis, delirium tremens, epi-
        lepsy or seizure disorders, and alcoholic blackouts.

1.163   Willoughby, Alan. "Helpful and Unhelpful Definitions."
        Chapter in The Alcohol Troubled Person: Known and Un-
        known, by Alan Willoughby, 45-63. Chicago, IL: Nel-
        son-Hall, Inc., 1979.

        There are many definitions of the word "alcoholic."
        There are definitions based on when a person drinks,
        where he drinks, with whom he drinks, and what he
        drinks. There are psychoanalytic definitions and Alco-
        holics Anonymous (AA) definitions.

1.164   Woeber, Karlheinz. "The Skin in Diagnosis of Alcohol-
        ism." Annals of the New York Academy of Sciences 252
        (1975): 292-295.

        A dermatologist elaborates on the effects of alcohol on
        the skin, and how this knowledge can be used in diagno-
        sing alcoholism. Author biographical information.

1.165   Wood, M.E. "Assessment of Chronic Alcoholism by Medi-
        cal Examination." New Zealand Medical Journal 99 (May
        14, 1986): 326-330.

        This research was carried out in Auckland, New Zealand
        and involved nearly 600 people admitted as patients to
        the Auckland Bridge Programme of the Salvation Army. A
        clinical examination of each patient and laboratory
        tests were used to study severity of alcoholic injury.

One aspect of this investigation was to examine the effectiveness of mean cell volume (MCV) and gamma glutamyl transpeptidase (GGT) in determining extent of chronic alcoholism. Author biographical information. Abstract. 3 tables. 1 figure. 11 references.

1.166   Woodman, Christopher. "A Reliability Study of an Automated Michigan Alcoholism Screening Test (MAST)." Dissertation Abstracts International 47: 2192B. Ph.D. dissertation, Florida Institute of Technology, 1985. Order No. DA8610404.

A computer administered version of the Michigan Alcoholism Screening Test (MAST) was found to be as reliable as a pencil and paper format.

1.167   Woodruff, Robert A., Jr., Paula J. Clayton, C. Robert Cloninger and Samuel B. Guze. "A Brief Method of Screening for Alcoholism." Diseases of the Nervous System 37 (1976): 434-435.

Criteria for alcoholism, frequency of symptoms of alcoholism, and alcoholics identified by report of excessive drinking. Author biographical information. 3 tables. 3 references.

1.168   Zabourek, Rothlyn P. "Identification of the Alcoholic in the Acute Care Setting." CCQ 8 (March 1986): 1-10.

Six topics: definitions and degree of the problem of alcoholism, signs of chemical dependence, process of assessment, defenses of the alcoholic, countering defenses, and intervention. This includes nine behavioral signs of chemical dependence, sixteen questions to ask the patient when obtaining his history of drinking, and twelve points to bear in mind regarding intervention. Author biographical information. 2 exhibits. 11 references.

2

Companies and Management

2.001   "Alcoholism." in <u>Understanding Personnel Management</u>,
by Thomas H. Stone, 453-455. Chicago, IL: Dryden Press,
1982.

Scope of the problem of employee alcoholism. Reasons why
managers can easily become alcoholics. Examples of successful alcoholism treatment progams in industry.

2.002   "Alcoholism Program Launched by Major Company." <u>Plant
Management and Engineering</u> 34 (November 1975): 7.

Employee alcoholism treatment program at Ford of Canada.

2.003   "Alcoholism Program Set Up by GM and UAW." <u>Automotive
Industries</u> 147 (July 15, 1972): 22.

An annoucement by the United Automobile Workers (UAW)
and General Motors (GM) to cooperate in the identification, referral, and follow-up treatment of GM employees
in the U.S., who are alcoholics.

2.004   "Alcoholism: Supervisors Are the Key." <u>Electrical
World</u> 195 (September 1981): 62.

Supervisors in electric utilities can help alcoholic employees by ensuring they receive proper treatment for
their alcoholism. Consolidated Edison Co. is mentioned
as having started its alcoholism program in the 1940s.

2.005   "Alcoholism Treatment Seen Cost-Effective by Kemper Executive." <u>Labor-Management Alcoholism Journal</u> 10 (January-February 1981): 165.

The comments of Dr. Gary Graham regarding the cost-benefit ratio of corporate alcoholism treatment programs.
Graham, Medical Director for the Kemper Group, spoke at
a meeting of the National Conference on Health Insurance.

2.006   Appelbaum, Steven H.   "Rescuing Time from the Bottle."
        Canadian Banker and ICB Review 89 (December 1982):   22-
        26.

        A look at the impact of alcoholism on the alcoholic em-
        ployee and his employer. Gives the economic impact of
        employee alcoholism on North American Rockwell Corp.,
        Gulf Canada Ltd., and the Illinois Bell Telephone Co.
        Lists ten indicators of employee alcoholism. Discusses
        at length the stages of alcoholism. Talks about the ten
        steps of an alcoholism counseling program. Author bio-
        graphical information. 3 sketches.

2.007   Arkin, Joseph. "The Problem Employee: The Alcoholic."
        PIMA Magazine 66 (February 1984):   15.

        Fifteen on-the-job drinking signs which characterize
        early or middle stage alcoholism. Also gives three ma-
        jor sources of unbiased information on treating alcohol-
        ism. The latter includes complete addresses.

2.008   Asma, Fern E. "Long-Term Experience with Rehabilitation
        of Alcoholic Employees." Chapter in Occupational Alco-
        holism Programs, edited by Richard L. Williams and Gene
        H. Moffat, 175-193. Springfield, IL: Charles C. Thom-
        as, Publisher, 1975.

        Rehabilitation of alcoholic employees at the Illinois
        Bell Telephone Co. The program was started in 1950.
        Areas covered by this chapter include: the extent of
        problem drinking, when problem drinking becomes a compa-
        ny problem, the Illinois Bell Telephone policy on prob-
        lem drinking, the role of the medical department, and
        program evaluation. 1 figure. 11 tables. 5 references.

2.009   "The Atlantic Richfield Program: The Right Man in the
        Right Place at the Right Time." Labor-Management Alco-
        holism Journal 6 (March-April 1977):   5-16.

        The Atlantic Richfield Co. (ARCO) began its employee al-
        coholism program (EAP) in 1974 with William G. Durkin as
        Employee Assistance Coordinator. This article includes
        excerpts from ARCO's policy on alcoholism and drug abuse.
        Company publications such as the ARCO Spark help promote
        the program. 5 photographs. 4 figures.

2.010   "Baltimore Group Starts Program." Labor-Management Alco-
        holism Journal 8 (March-April 1979):   198.

        The Greater Baltimore Committee will assist up to 1500
        business organizations in the Baltimore area, in the es-
        tablishment of employee alcoholism programs (EAPs).

2.011   Barry, Lawrence M. "Industrial Alcoholism Programs: The
        Problem, The Program, The Professional." Family

Coordinator 25 (January 1976):   65-72.

History of industrial alcoholism programs. Abstract.
Author biographical information. 1 figure. 10 references.

2.012   Beach, Dale S.   "Alcoholism."   in Personnel: The Management of People at Work, by Dale S. Beach, Third Edition, 746-749. New York, NY: Macmillan Publishing
Co., Inc., 1975.

Lever Brothers, American Motors, and Merrill Lynch are
three of numerous companies which have alcoholism control programs for alcoholic employees. A policy statement, union cooperation, education, training, and professional services are the main elements in an alcoholism control program.

2.013   Bealer, John D.   "Hiring Recovered Alcoholics: A Policy That Pays." Labor-Management Alcoholism Journal 7
(November-December 1977):   20-21.

States why recovered alcoholics should be hired. Cites
the example of a bank with a policy for eight years of
employing recovered alcoholics. Only about 2% of the
recovered alcoholics that were hired were terminated
because of relapse drinking. Author biographical information. 1 photograph.

2.014   Beaumont, P.B. and S.J. Allsop. "An Industrial Alcohol
Policy: The Characteristics of Worker Success." British Journal of Addiction 79 (1984):   315-318.

Forty-eight company employees received treatment for alcohol problems. Fourteen of the employees voluntarily
sought help. Thirty-four were referred by the employer.
Self-referral was associated with poor treatment outcome compared to employer referral. Author biographical information. Abstract. 3 tables. 18 references.

2.015   Beeman, Don R.   "Is the Social Drinker Killing Your Company?" Business Horizons 28 (January-February 1985):
54-58.

It is not alcoholics, but light-to-moderate drinkers who
can constitute the greatest employee problem for employers. Problems with alcoholics at work tend to be quite
obvious. The impaired intellectual ability of light-to-
moderate drinkers is often not apparent. Author biographical information. 3 tables. 1 illustration.

2.016   Black, Paul V.   "Employee Alcoholism on the Burlington
Railroad, 1876-1902." Journal of the West 17 (October
1978):   5-11.

Employee alcoholism was a serious problem among railroad workers in the nineteenth century. This article discusses the extent of the problem and attempts to effectively deal with it. Drinking by rank and file employees and by executives is examined. A statement describing the Burlington Railroad's policy on drinking is included. 4 photographs. Author biographical information. 37 notes.

2.017   Booth, Derrick. "If an Alcoholic Was Running Your Works, Would You Know?" Engineer 238 (May 2, 1974): 28-29.

Twenty ways to spot an alcoholic employee. 1 cartoon illustration.

2.018   Bower, Catherine D. "Alcoholism: Industry's $9 Billion Headache." Personnel Administrator 20 (January 1975): 32-35.

How companies deal with employee alcoholism. The Allen-Bradley Co., McDonnell Douglas, Allis-Chalmers, Consolidated Edison, Bethlehem Steel, and Du Pont are some of the companies. Companies are discovering they can save money by rehabilitating alcoholic employees. The value and importance of union cooperation is stressed.

2.019   Brent, J. Ford. "A Semantic Trap." Labor-Management Alcoholism Journal 10 (January-February 1981): 146-147.

Comments on the expression "job threat" and employee alcoholism programs (EAPs). Author biographical information.

2.020   Brisolara, Ashton. "Approaching the Troubled Employee." Chapter in The Alcoholic Employee: A Handbook of Useful Guidelines, by Ashton Brisolara, 107-124. New York, NY: Human Sciences Press, 1979.

A twenty-question Employee Work Performance Scale and the Ladder of Employee Deterioration can help identify the employee who has an alcohol or drug problem. The supervisor should be understanding, fair, pleasant, kind, sincere, and firm. He should not lecture, scold, or lose his temper. 1 chart. 2 references.

2.021   Brisolara, Ashton. "Case Histories." Chapter in The Alcoholic Employee: A Handbook of Useful Guidelines, by Ashton Brisolara, 125-136. New York, NY: Human Sciences Press, 1979.

Seven case histories about alcoholic employees.

2.022   Brisolara, Ashton. "Company Educational Projects." Chapter in The Alcoholic Employee: A Handbook of Useful Guidelines, by Ashton Brisolara, 137-145. New York, NY:

Human Sciences Press, 1979.

Audiovisual aids, such as films, and also payroll in-
serts, can help make company alcoholism and drug abuse
programs more successful. A list of sixteen films is
included.

2.023   Brisolara, Ashton. "Industrial Alcoholism." Chapter
in The Alcoholic Employee: A Handbook of Useful Guidelines, by Ashton Brisolara, 11-33. New York, NY: Human Sciences Press, 1979.

Allis-Chalmers, Consolidated Edison, Great Northern
Railway, Detroit Edison, Du Pont, Minnesota Mining, and
Peoples' Light and Coke Co. are examples of companies
which have industrial alcoholism programs, and which
have found their programs to be profitable financially
and in other ways. 1 chart. 6 references.

2.024   Brisolara, Ashton. "Industrial Alternatives." Chapter
in The Alcoholic Employee: A Handbook of Useful Guidelines, by Ashton Brisolara, 71-82. New York, NY: Human Sciences Press, 1979.

Explains the rationale of employee alcoholism programs
(EAPs), the alternatives to not having a program, employees as investments, what constitutes a program, and
legal considerations.

2.025   Brisolara, Ashton. "Policy." Chapter in The Alcoholic
Employee: A Handbook of Useful Guidelines, by Ashton
Brisolara, 83-94. New York, NY: Human Sciences Press,
1979.

Nineteen points to include in a company alcoholism policy. An example of a nine-point policy on alcoholism and
drug abuse is also included. 4 charts.

2.026   Brisolara, Ashton. "Referral." Chapter in The Alcoholic Employee: A Handbook of Useful Guidelines, by Ashton
Brisolara, 146-155. New York, NY: Human Sciences Press,
1979.

The medical profession, counselors and social workers,
the clergy, and Alcoholics Anonymous (AA) can help the
alcoholic employee.

2.027   Brisolara, Ashton. "Resources." Chapter in The Alcoholic Employee: A Handbook of Useful Guidelines, by Ashton
Brisolara, 156-158. New York, NY: Human Sciences Press,
1979.

Thirty-nine local, state, and national sources of information about alcoholism and drug abuse.

2.028   Brisolara, Ashton. "The Supervisory Force." Chapter
         in The Alcoholic Employee: A Handbook of Useful Guide-
         lines, by Ashton Brisolara, 95-106. New York, NY: Hu-
         man Sciences Press, 1979.

         Outlines thirty-two, on-the-job clues which indicate an
         alcoholic or drug-abusing employee and which supervi-
         sors should bear in mind. Ten of the clues: absentee-
         ism, unusual excuses, mood changes, red or bleary eyes,
         loud talking, suspiciousness, tremors, excessive ner-
         vousness, flushed face, and resentfulness. Also listed
         are eight things to discuss at supervisory staff meet-
         ings in order to attain an effective alcoholism program.
         1 chart.

2.029   "The Brooklyn Union Gas Program: The Easy Road to Super-
         visory Cooperation." Labor-Management Alcoholism Jour-
         nal 6 (September-October 1976): 5-19.

         Joseph Rodriguez, a former alcoholic and employee of the
         Brooklyn Union Gas Co., was instrumental in establishing
         the Alcoholics Assistance Program at Union Gas. 6 pho-
         tographs. 2 figures.

2.030   Brubaker, Warren W. "Alcoholism in Industry." Occupa-
         tional Health Nursing 25 (February 1977): 7-10.

         This paper was presented on October 16, 1976 in Hershey,
         Pennsylvania at a seminar about the troubled employee.
         The seminar was sponsored by the Central Pennsylvania
         AOHN (Association of Occupational Health Nurses). In-
         cludes a twenty-question alcoholism questionnaire. Au-
         thor biographical information. 1 figure.

2.031   Buckton, Ray. "Alcoholism and Industry." Chapter in
         Alcohol Related Problems: Room for Manoeuvre, edited by
         Neville Krasner, J.S. Madden and Robin J. Walker, 37-40.
         New York, NY: John Wiley and Sons, Ltd., 1984.

         Alcoholism and industry in Britain, union and management
         efforts to deal with it, economic, social, and medical
         costs of alcoholism. This chapter was first presented
         as a paper at the Fifth International Conference on Al-
         cohol Related Problems, Liverpool, April 1981.

2.032   Burton, Wayne N., Paul R. Eggum and Phillip J. Keller.
         "'High Cost' Employees in an Occupational Alcoholism
         Program: A Preliminary Report." Journal of Occupational
         Medicine 23 (1981): 259-262.

         The Health Counseling Program at International Harvester
         Co. This program was established for alcoholic employees
         in 1975. The focus of this article is on those employees
         who received more than $1000.00 in medical or disability

payments during a one-year period. Author biographical information. Abstract. 6 tables. 12 references.

2.033   "Business Drinking: A 'Health Hazard.'" U.S. News and World Report 72 (March 13, 1972): 70-71.

Interview with Dr. Harry J. Johnson, Chairman, Medical Board, Life Extension Institute. 1 photograph.

2.034   Byers, William R. and John C. Quinn. "Alcoholism as a Major Focus of EAPs." Chapter in The Human Resources Management Handbook: Principles and Practice of Employee Assistance Programs, edited by Samuel H. Klarreich, James L. Francek and C. Eugene Moore, 370-380. New York, NY: Praeger Publishers, 1985.

Among key issues dealt with: the prevalence, scope, and costs of alcoholism and alcohol misuse; the rationale for a major focus on alcoholism; and the types of employee problems identified by employee assistance programs (EAPs). In the U.S., the annual cost of alcoholism to society is estimated to be $120 billion. 1 table. 31 references.

2.035   Carlile, Harold E. "Positive Counseling for the Employee with an Alcohol Problem." Thrust 11 (March-April 1982): 38-39.

Describes how to positively confront, through three meetings, the alcoholic employee. Author biographical information.

2.036   Chopra, Khem S., Donald A. Preston and Lowell W. Gerson. "The Effect of Constructive Coercion on the Rehabilitative Process: A Study of the Employed Alcoholics in an Alcoholism Treatment Program." Journal of Occupational Medicine 21 (1979): 749-752.

Based on a paper presented at the Canadian Addiction Foundation in Winnipeg, Manitoba in July 1977. Author biographical information. Abstract. 5 tables. 14 references.

2.037   Chruden, Herbert J. and Arthur W. Sherman, Jr. "The Problem of Alcoholism." in Personnel Management, by Herbert J. Chruden and Arthur W. Sherman, Jr., Fifth Edition, 313. Cincinnati, OH: South-Western Publishing Co., 1976.

Overview of industrial alcoholism.

2.038   Cockram, Frank. "Winning the Battle of the Bottle." CTM: The Human Element 15 (December 1982): 14-16.

A number of employers in Canada have programs which

assist the alcoholic employee. Dominion Foundries and
Steel, the University of Guelph, Massey-Ferguson, the
Toronto Transit Commission, and Ontario Hydro are five
such employers. This article also lists sixteen key
components of employee assistance programs (EAPs) and
describes three treatment facilities for alcoholics in
Toronto: the Pinewood Treatment Centre, the Donwood Institute, and Renascent House. Author biographical information.

2.039   Collins, Robert. "Drinking on the Job." Imperial Oil
        Review 57, No. 2 (1973): 2-7.

        Imperial Oil, Eaton's, Simpsons, General Motors (GM),
        Kodak, and the Royal Bank are some of the companies in
        Canada which have employee alcoholism programs (EAPs).
        The Donwood Foundation and the May Street Clinic, both
        in Toronto, provide treatment for alcoholics. Dr. Clif-
        ford Preece, of Imperial Oil's medical department, com-
        ments on alcoholism. 3 photographs.

2.040   Combs-Orme, Terri, John R. Taylor and Lee N. Robins.
        "Occupational Prestige and Mortality in Black and White
        Alcoholics." Journal of Studies on Alcohol 46 (1985):
        443-446.

        The subjects in this study were Black and White alcohol-
        ics in the St. Louis, Missouri area. The total number
        of subjects in the sample was 1289. Black alcoholics
        were significantly younger at death than were White al-
        coholics. Occupational prestige was divided into high,
        medium, and low categories. Author biographical infor-
        mation. Abstract. 3 tables. 19 references.

2.041   "Coverage for Alcoholism Treatment Is Cutting Employer
        Disability Cost." Business Insurance 10 (November 15,
        1976): 62.

        Economic Laboratory, Inc. of St. Paul, Minnesota and
        Scovill Manufacturing Co. of Waterbury, Connecticut are
        two companies with alcoholism treatment programs. These
        programs are successful in more than one way. They have
        a high rehabilitation success rate and save the compa-
        nies money.

2.042   Cummings, Paul W. "Handling the Alcoholic Employee."
        Training and Development Journal 29 (February 1975): 42-
        44.

        A six-point guide for industrial training personnel--in
        small, medium or large companies--to use in handling al-
        coholic employees. Author biographical information. 4
        references.

2.043   Cunnick, William R., Jr. and Edgar P. Marchesini. "The

Program for Alcoholism at Metropolitan Life." Chapter
in Alcoholism and Its Treatment in Industry, edited by
Carl J. Schramm, 82-90. Baltimore, MD: Johns Hopkins
University Press, 1977.

The focus of this chapter is on the history, policy, and
objectives of the alcoholism program at Metropolitan
Life. This company issued in 1960 its written policy on
alcoholism. This chapter includes seven guidelines for
supervisors to use in dealing with employee behavioral
problems, and ten criteria for evaluating inpatient rehabilitation centers. A table gives statistics about
the alcoholism program for the years 1961-1972. 1 table.

2.044   Daghestani, Amin N., Peter Barglow, Robert R.J. Hilker
        and Fern E. Asma. "The Supervisor's Role with the
        Problem Drinker Employee." Journal of Occupational Med-
        icine 18 (1976): 85-90.

        The authors did this study at the Illinois Bell Tele-
        phone Co., a public utility company which employs 41,000
        people. Problem drinker employees and supervisors took
        part in the research. Questionnaires and interviews
        were used. The study took place between summer 1974 and
        spring 1975. Author biographical information. 13 ta-
        bles. 2 figures. 27 references.

2.045   Davies, John B. "Reported Alcohol Consumption, and At-
        titudes of Managerial and Non-Managerial Employees, in a
        Study of Five Industries on Clydeside." British Journal
        on Alcohol and Alcoholism 13 (Winter 1978): 160-169.

        This investigation took place in Scotland and involved
        576 employees--444 men and 132 women. These individuals
        were employed by five employers: a brewery, a shipyard,
        a motor vehicle manufacturer, a manufacturer of propul-
        sion units, and a regional council department. Each
        member of the sample was interviewed and filled in two
        self-completion questionnaires. Author biographical in-
        formation. Abstract. 3 figures. 2 tables. 8 refer-
        ences.

2.046   Denenberg, Tia Schneider and R.V. Denenberg. "The Bos-
        ton Gas Program." in Alcohol and Drugs: Issues in the
        Workplace, by Tia Schneider Denenberg and R.V. Denenberg,
        51-52. Washington, DC: Bureau of National Affairs, Inc.,
        1983.

        Rehabilitation of alcoholic employees at the Boston Gas
        Co.

2.047   Dimas, George C. "The Foundation of an Effective Pro-
        gram: A Written Policy on Alcoholism." Labor-Management
        Alcoholism Journal 6 (March-April 1977): 22-23.

States that a written policy on alcoholism must address
at least nine important questions. A written policy,
furthermore, fosters good employee and good public relations. This has been evidenced in the alcoholism
policies of companies like General Motors (GM) and Bethlehem Steel. Author biographical information. 1 photograph.

2.048   Duckert, Fanny. "Industrial Alcohol Programs in Norway." Chapter in Alcohol Problems in Employment, edited
by Brian D. Hore and Martin A. Plant, 161-172. London:
Croom Helm Ltd., 1981.

The AKAN Program is one of several programs which combat industrial alcoholism in Norway. This program--AKAN
is the acronym for the Committee of Industry and Trade--
began in 1963. The ISO Groups, based on a Danish program, began in Oslo in 1974. The Valo Project is a third
program. 1 figure.

2.049   Dunkin, William S. "The Invisible Disease: Alcoholism
in the Workplace." Public Welfare 41 (Winter 1983): 23-
27.

One example of the identification of alcoholics in the
workplace was in Lees Summit, Missouri, a suburb of Kansas City. An employee alcoholism program (EAP) revealed
that over 10% of the town's employees were alcoholics.
An inset section entitled "Savings" states how the Union
Pacific Railroad, New York Transit Authority, and General
Motors (GM) saved money by having employee alcoholism
programs (EAPs). 3 photographs. Author biographical information.

2.050   Dunkin, William S. "Policies in the United States."
Chapter in Alcohol Problems in Employment, edited by
Brian D. Hore and Martin A. Plant, 144-160. London:
Croom Helm Ltd., 1981.

The first employee alcoholism program (EAP) in the U.S.
was established in 1942 at E.I. du Pont de Nemours Co. i
Wilmington, Delaware. Despite the relatively high success rate of treating alcoholic employees, and despite
the fact it is more economical for companies to rehabili
tate than it is to dismiss these individuals, extremely
few companies have employee alcoholism programs (EAPs).
Companies generally do not want to admit they have these
problems. Myths and stigma about alcoholism persist.

2.051   Dunn, Earl V., Stephen Kandel and John Hilditch. "Signs
and Symptoms in Male Alcoholics." Canadian Journal of
Public Health 76 (September-October 1985): 308-311.

Nearly 500 male alcoholics--most of them referred for
treatment by industry, and most of them residing within

fifty miles of metropolitan Toronto, Ontario--were the
subjects of research. The authors investigated: the
pattern of drinking by the type of alcoholic beverage
consumed, family and medical history by type of alcoholic beverage consumed, past health by type of beverage consumed, signs and symptoms by type of beverage
consumed, patterns of drinking by palpable liver, medical and family history by palpable liver, past health
by palpable liver, and signs and symptoms by palpable
liver. Author biographical information. English abstract. French abstract. 8 tables. 6 references.

2.052   "Du Pont Hailed for First Alcoholism Program." Labor-
        Management Alcoholism Journal 7 (September-October
        1977): 29-30.

        The National Council on Alcoholism (NCA) awarded a spe-
        cial commendation to E.I. du Pont de Nemours and Co.,
        in recognition of the company's employee alcoholism
        treatment program. Du Pont veiwed alcoholism as a dis-
        ease as early as the 1940s--long before the American
        Medical Association (AMA) offcially recognized alcohol-
        ism as an illness. 1 photograph.

2.053   "The Eastman Kodak Program: A Favorable Climate." La-
        bor-Management Alcoholism Newsletter 2 (November-Decem-
        ber 1972): 1-15.

        How the employee alcoholism program (EAP) at the East-
        man Kodak Co. works. 3 photographs. 2 illustrations

2.054   Edwards, Mark R. and J. Ruth Sproull. "Confronting Al-
        coholism through Team Evaluation." Business Horizons
        29 (May-June 1986): 78-83.

        The Team Evaluation and Management System (TEAMS) can be
        used to confront alcoholics in the workplace. TEAMS is
        preferrable to traditional methods of appraising employ-
        ees because traditional methods give supervisors disin-
        centives for confronting the alcoholic worker. TEAMS is
        a peer-supplemented appraisal process. Ten steps to
        follow in implementing TEAMS are included. Author bio-
        graphical information. 11 footnotes. 2 illustrations.

2.055   "The Ex-Drunk's One-Martini Lunch." Economist 275
        (April 12, 1980): 18.

        Executive alcoholism and its treatment--particularly at
        Fenwick Hall, a mansion in South Carolina, where alco-
        holic executives are rehabilitated. Also discussed are
        remarks by Dr. Morris Chafetz, the first director of the
        National Institute on Alcohol Abuse and Alcoholism
        (NIAAA). Dr. Chafetz established Fenwick Hall.

2.056   Fennell, Mary L., Miriam B. Rodin and Glenda K. Kantor.

"Problems in the Work Setting, Drinking, and Reasons
for Drinking." Social Forces 60 (September 1981):
114-132.

A national sample of U.S. workers was used to test two
hypotheses by University of Illinois researchers. The
researchers learned that any one of eight different
work-setting problems were likely associated with a
worker's reason for drinking. The reasons were: not
enough information, cannot see results, not enough time,
conflicting demands, promotions unfair, no help from
supervisor, no help from co-workers, or co-workers in-
competent. Author biographical information. Abstract.
4 tables. 9 notes. 65 references.

2.057   Fillmore, Kaye Middleton. "Research as a Handmaiden of
        Policy: An Appraisal of Estimates of Alcoholism and Its
        Cost in the Workplace." Journal of Public Health Policy
        5 (March 1984): 40-64.

        Compares the Temperance Movement and alcohol in the
        workplace to the Modern Alcoholism Movement then ex-
        amines the loss to business and industry attributed to
        the alcoholic. 75 references.

2.058   "Film Aims at Top Management." Labor-Management Alco-
        holism Journal 6 (January-February 1977): 19 and 22.

        "To Meet a Need" is a nine-minute film for the top-level
        executive market. The film is about employee alcoholism
        and employee alcoholism programs (EAPs). 1 photograph.

2.059   Fine, Michelle, Sheila H. Akabas and Susan Bellinger.
        "Cultures of Drinking: A Workplace Perspective." So-
        cial Work 27 (September 1982): 436-440.

        How industrial social workers can, in the workplace,
        help change a culture-of-drinking environment into a
        culture-of-sobriety environment. Author biographical
        information. Abstract. 25 notes and references.

2.060   Follmann, Joseph F., Jr. "Effects on the Business Com-
        munity." Chapter in Alcoholics and Business: Prob-
        lems, Costs, Solutions, by Joseph F. Follmann, Jr., 78-
        94. New York, NY: AMACOM, 1976.

        Four sections comprise this chapter: alcoholism in in-
        dustry, the cost to American business, employers' atti-
        tudes, and the attitude of organized labor. 2 tables.
        23 notes.

2.061   Follmann, Joseph F., Jr. "Some Accomplishments to
        Date." Chapter in Alcoholics and Business: Problems,
        Costs, Solutions, by Joseph F. Follmann, Jr., 159-176.
        New York, NY: AMACOM, 1976.

Lists employers who claim success in rehabilitating alcoholic employees. Two of these employers are Standard
Oil of Oregon and the Caterpillar Tractor Co. Also
lists alcohol control programs which are cost-effective.
One of these is at the Scovill Manufacturing Co.; another is at Illinois Bell Telephone. 3 tables. 39 notes.

2.062 Follmann, Joseph F., Jr. "What Can Be Done?" Chapter
in Alcoholics and Business: Problems, Costs, Solutions,
by Joseph F. Follmann, Jr., 119-158. New York, NY:
AMACOM, 1976.

Begins by discussing what is being done by employers
about employee alcoholism. Then talks about specific
employment-centered alcoholism control programs. This
is followed by information on how to set up an alcoholism control program. Three other sections complete
this chapter: the role of private insurers, the problems
of small businesses, and where to get help in establishing an employee alcoholism program (EAP). 1 table. 23
notes.

2.063 Forcier, Michael W. "Labor Force Behavior of Alcoholics: A Review." International Journal of the Addictions 20 (1985): 253-268.

Compares three viewpoints pertaining to alcoholics. Reasons are given for each viewpoint. For example, the
first viewpoint involved biased samples of alcoholic psychotics and arrested public drunks. Author biographical
information. Abstract. 4 tables. 3 notes. 27 references.

2.064 "Former Executive Sues Ford for Losses Due to Alcohol."
Industry Week 186 (August 4, 1975): 11-12.

John R. Brennan was formerly chairman and managing director of Ford Motor Co. (Switzerland) S.A. He took
early retirement in 1970 and subsequently sued his former employer for $1.3 million. Brennan claimed the na-
ture of his work led to his alcoholism.

2.065 Francis, G. James and Gene Milbourn, Jr. "Alcoholism."
in Human Behavior in the Work Environment: A Managerial
Perspective, by G. James Francis and Gene Milbourn, Jr.,
125-130. Santa Monica, CA: Goodyear Publishing Co.,
Inc., 1980.

Views alcoholism as a disease with many causes and costs,
states how to identify the alcoholic employee, and discusses programs to reduce alcoholism.

2.066 Gallagher, Joan M. "Alcoholic Executives: Issues and
Treatment Strategies." Labor-Management Alcoholism
Journal 9 (July-August 1979): 42-44.

Case studies associated with the Boston College Occupational Alcohol and Drug Training Program. Five reasons why alcoholic executives are different from other
company alcoholics. A twelve-point profile of the alcoholic executive. Eight points about confronting this
type of alcoholic are listed. Author biographical information.

2.067   Geneen, Harold. "Not Alcoholism--Egotism." Chapter in
Managing, by Harold Geneen, 173-186. New York, NY:
Avon Books, 1984.

Harold Geneen, the former head of ITT (International
Telephone and Telegraph), talks about alcohol abuse in
industry, and how he dealt with this problem when ITT
staff abused alcohol. He comments on the personal costs
to the afflicted employee and the economic costs to the
corporation.

2.068   "General Dynamics Pomona Division Uses 'Low Profile'
Approach." Labor-Management Alcoholism Journal 6 (November-December 1976): 3-17.

The work of Charles A. Poulson, Jr., in administering
the General Dynamics Pomona (California) Division employee assistance program (EAP), which was announced in
February 1975. Over 40% of referrals to the program involved alcoholism. 5 photographs. 7 figures.

2.069   "German Company Encourages Rehabilitation of Alcoholic-
s." Management Review 71 (April 1982): 41.

Gisela Langensee planned and developed an employee alcoholism program (EAP) at Voith, Inc., a German company
that manufactures engine parts.

2.070   Gibson, W. David. "They're Bringing Problem Drinkers
Out of the Closet." Chemical Week 123 (November 15,
1978): 85-86, 88 and 91.

Representatives from industry--Dow Chemical, Union Carbide, and Kaiser Aluminum and Chemical are three exam-
ples--talk about industrial alcoholism. There is also a
list of seventeen indicators of employee alcoholism. 1
photograph.

2.071   Glaser, Frederick B., Stephanie W. Greenberg and Morris
Barrett. "Industrial Programs in Pennsylvania." Chapter in A Systems Approach to Alcohol Treatment, by Frederick B. Glaser, Stephanie W. Greenberg and Morris Barrett, 153-163. Toronto: Addiction Research Foundation,
1978.

Industrial alcoholism programs in the Philadelphia area
are described, as are program design and the supervisor

as a key person in program success. Also covered are:
the initial interview, a second interview with the problem employee, implementation of the rehabilitation program, disciplinary action--if needed, and continued deterioration of job performance. A guide for supervisors
for identifying the alcoholic employee and leadership
initiatives from governmental and private sectors are
described. 2 tables. 5 references.

2.072   Goodall, Kenneth. "Alcoholism Recovery Pays Off for
        Oldsmobile." Psychology Today 9 (September 1975): 85
        and 87.

        Reports on the success of the voluntary Employee Alco-
        holism Recovery Program at the Oldsmobile Division of
        General Motors Corp. in Lansing, Michigan. Two Olds-
        mobile employees, Ross P. Alander and Thomas J. Camp-
        bell, evaluated the program.

2.073   Goodwin, Rowland. "The Drink Factor." in Stress at
        Work: A Study of a Growing Problem in Industry, by
        Rowland Goodwin, 109. London: Chester House Publica-
        tions, 1976.

        Alcohol abuse in British industry.

2.074   Googins, Bradley and Norman R. Kurtz. "Discriminating
        Participating and Nonparticipating Supervisors in Oc-
        cupational Alcoholism Programs." Journal of Drug Is-
        sues 11 (1981): 199-216.

        A study about supervisors and occupational alcoholism
        programs (OAPs) in a company with over 40,000 person-
        nel. Two groups of supervisors were compared--refer-
        ring supervisors, and nonreferring supervisors. Refer-
        ring supervisors referred alcoholic employees for treat-
        ment. Nonreferring supervisors did not make referrals.
        Discriminators or barriers that prevent referral were
        identified. Age, length of time in position, and years
        in the company were three discriminators/barriers iden-
        tified. Four hundred and fifty-seven supervisors took
        part in this study. Author biographical information.
        Abstract. 5 tables. 2 figures. 2 notes. 18 refer-
        ences.

2.075   Googins, Bradley and Norman R. Kurtz. "Factors Inhibit-
        ing Supervisory Referrals to Occupational Alcoholism In-
        tervention Programs." Journal of Studies on Alcohol 41
        (1980): 1196-1208.

        Attitudes, job satisfaction, and labor-management rela-
        tionships are some of the factors inhibiting supervisory
        referrals to occupational alcoholism intervention pro-
        grams. Abstract. Author biographical information. 33
        references.

2.076   Goshen, Charles E.   "Special Management Problems: The
        Problem Drinker."   Chapter in The Management of Deci-
        sions and the Decisions of Management, by Charles E.
        Goshen, 247-258. New York, NY: Vantage Press, 1975.

        Nature and scope of the problem of alcoholic workers in
        industry, their detection, utilization, and the role of
        the employer in rehabilitating these people.

2.077   Grayzel, Estherann F.   "Employee Assistance: Estab-
        lishing and Maintaining a Program in a Diverse Corpo-
        rate Setting." Journal of Occupational Medicine 24
        (1982):   614-616.

        A medical director and the establishment of an employ-
        ee assistance program (EAP) in a corporate setting--
        General Foods Corp. Like many EAPs, this program ini-
        tially dealt with alcoholic employees. The program was
        later modified to include nonalcoholic problems. Author
        biographical information. 2 figures.

2.078   Guida, Miriam.   "The Occupational Health Nurse's Role
        in the Corporate Alcoholism Program." Occupational
        Health Nursing 24 (March 1976): 22-24.

        Includes a section on alcoholism training for the occu-
        pational health nurse. Author biographical information.
        1 photograph. 12 references.

2.079   Guida, Miriam A.   "OHNs Are in the Best Position to Help
        Workers Fight Alcoholism." Occupational Health and
        Safety 47 (September-October 1978):   48-52.

        Role of occupational health nurses in the early inter-
        vention and treatment of alcoholic employees. Author
        biographical information. 3 photographs. 6 references.

2.080   Guidelines for Establishing a Company Program." Nurs-
        ing 75 5 (December 1975):   50.

        Lists in point form eight guidelines for setting up for
        employees a company, alcoholic rehabilitation program.

2.081   "The 'Half-Man.'" Toronto Board of Trade Journal 66
        (June 1976):   50-51.

        Reports on a one-day symposium on alcoholism held in To-
        ronto, Ontario. The symposium was sponsored by Ontario
        Blue Cross and attracted 200 corporate delegates. Gwyl
        Jones (Du Pont of Canada) and C.R. Lunn (General Motors
        of Canada) were two of the delegates. 1 photograph.

2.082   "He Cures Kennecott's People Problems." Business Week
        (April 15, 1972):   113-114.

Otto F. Jones works for the Kennecott Copper Corp. in Salt Lake City, Utah and assists employees who have a variety of problems, including alcoholism. Jones is head of Insight, a program that provides confidential help for Kennecott employees. Unions are among the strongest supporters of Insight. 3 photographs.

2.083 "Health Conservation Is Keynote at Metropolitan Life." Labor-Management Alcoholism Newsletter 2 (January-February 1973): 1-7.

Metropolitan Life established, in the late 1940s, an employee alcoholism program (EAP). The program is administered by William R. Cunnick, Jr., John B. Cromie, and Edgar P. Marchesini. 3 photographs. 2 figures.

2.084 "A Helping Hand from the Consortium." Report on Business Magazine 3 (September 1986): 74.

The London Employee Assistance Consortium (LEAC) in London, Ontario was established in 1976. John Labatt Ltd., Kellogg Salada Canada Inc., General Motors of Canada Ltd., 3M Canada Inc., Canadian International Paper Inc., and Union Gas created LEAC. Alcoholism is only one type of problem dealt with by LEAC's staff. The annual LEAC budget is $250,000.00. 1 photograph.

2.085 Hemmett, Gordon L. "What Can Supervisors Do about Alcoholic Subordinates?" Supervisory Management 17 (December 1972): 13-18.

Defines alcoholism, describes its progression as an illness, talks about psychological blocks to rehabilitation, outlines the use of friendly persuasion in helping the alcoholic employee, discusses the alcoholic's denial there is anything wrong with him, and concludes by stating what should be done when friendly persuasion fails. The preceding is based on experiences at the Eastman Kodak Co. Author biographical information.

2.086 Hendrickson, Jane E. "The Alcoholic Employee: How the Nurse Can Help." Nursing 75 5 (December 1975): 46-47 and 49-50.

Role of the industrial nurse in recognizing, confronting, and helping the alcoholic employee. 1 illustration.

2.087 Herbert, Henry R. "Alcoholism: The Supervisor's Role in Rehabilitation." Supervisory Management 20 (December 1975): 7-14.

Fictitious dialogue between a company spokesman, explaining a company's policy on alcoholism, and supervisors who have questions and comments regarding the

policy. Author biographical information. 1 illustration.

2.088   Hernandez, M. Jean and Rebecca L. Hamilton. "An Educational Approach to Employee Problem Drinking." <u>Jour-
nal of the College and University Personnel Association</u>
35 (Summer 1984): 4-7.

Educational methods employers can use to help prevent
or minimize employee alcohol dependency. Includes a
list of organizations which provide alcoholism literature. 12 footnotes.

2.089   Herold, David M. and Edward J. Conlon. "Work Factors
as Potential Causal Agents of Alcohol Abuse." <u>Journal
of Drug Issues</u> 11 (1981): 337-356.

These authors contend that evidence demonstrating that
a person's work may contribute to alcohol abuse is
scarce. Author biographical information. Abstract. 3
figures. 33 references.

2.090   Heyman, Margaret M. "Referral to Alcoholism Programs
in Industry: Coercion, Confrontation and Choice." <u>Jour-
nal of Studies on Alcohol</u> 37 (1976): 900-907.

Coercion was found to be an effective method of convincing alcoholic employees to seek treatment for their alcoholism. Treated employees demonstrated a high degree
of work improvement. The employees studied participated
in industrial alcoholism programs in New York City. Abstract. Author biographical information. 6 footnotes.
6 references.

2.091   Hilker, Robert R.J., Fern E. Asma and Raymond L. Eggert.
"A Company-Sponsored Alcoholic Rehabilitation Program:
Ten Year Evaluation." <u>Journal of Occupational Medicine</u>
14 (1972): 769-772.

The Illinois Bell Telephone Co. established in 1951 a
treatment program for alcoholic employees. The program
was not viewed enthusiastically, in its early days, by
either management or employees. An evaluation of the
program, based on more than 400 employees, indicated the
program was very successful. The company, employees,
family, and society in general benefited when, for example, job efficiency was increased, sickness disability
decreased, and off-the-job and on-the-job accidents were
reduced. This paper was presented at the Fifty-Seventh
Annual Meeting, Industrial Medical Association, Philadelphia, April 19, 1972. Author biographical information.
16 tables.

2.092   Hore, B.D. "Alcohol and Alcoholism: The Impact on
Work." in <u>Alcoholism: New Knowledge and New Responses</u>,

edited by Griffith Edwards and Marcus Grant, 244-250.
Baltimore, MD: University Park Press, 1977.

Examines: the effect of alcohol on physiological and
psychological variables associated with work performance, work problems arising from alcohol abuse in industry, and the detection of alcohol abuse in industry
and its management. 15 references.

2.093   Horn, Jack. "Corporate Alcoholism--What Makes a Good
        Company Program." Psychology Today 9 (September 1975):
        87.

        The Corporate Headquarters Alcoholism Project (CHAP) be-
        gan, in 1975, to study alcoholism treatment programs
        used by corporations based in New York. Money for CHAP
        was obtained from the National Institute on Alcohol
        Abuse and Alcoholism (NIAAA). Includes address where
        to write for more information.

2.094   "How Business Grapples with Problem of the Drinking
        Worker." U.S. News and World Report 77 (July 15, 1974):
        75-76.

        Problem drinkers cost American industry $15 billion an-
        nually. Although many companies have been reluctant to
        establish rehabilitation programs for alcoholic employ-
        ees, that trend has been changing in favor of such pro-
        grams. General Motors (GM), for example, has alcoholism
        committees in 111 plants. James S. Kemper, Jr., Pres-
        ident, Kemper Insurance and Financial Companies, states
        that the prospect of losing a job is the alcoholic em-
        ployee's strongest motivator to accept treatment. 1 pho-
        tograph. 1 table.

2.095   "How to Keep Your Executives on the Road--and the Wagon."
        Canadian Business 54 (March 1981): 150-151.

        Overview of business travel and alcohol: symptoms of
        drinking problems, medical consequences, profile of the
        traveling alcoholic, how to help and where to get help.
        An inset section is entitled "Setting Up a Sober Hospi-
        tality Suite." 1 photograph.

2.096   Hughes, J.P.W. "Alcoholism in Industry." Medicine,
        Science and the Law 15, No. 1 (1975): 22-27.

        A paper presented to the Annual General Meeting, Brit-
        ish Academy of Forensic Sciences, London, June 14, 1974.
        Author biographical information. 13 tables. 9 refer-
        ences.

2.097   Husbands, Walter T. "Programming in a National General
        Merchandise Retail Chain: The J.C. Penney Company Ex-
        perience." Labor-Management Alcoholism Journal 7

(May-June 1978):   28-38.

The employee alcoholism program (EAP) at J.C. Penney
Co. was launched nationally in 1977. Its formal name
is the "Job Performance Action Program." J.C. Penney
employs 185,000 men and women in the U.S. Author biographical information. 1 photograph.

2.098 Illinois Bell Telephone Co. Medical Department. "Rehabilitation of the Problem Drinker." in Management of
Human Resources, by Edwin L. Miller, Elmer H. Burack
and Maryann H. Albrecht, 420-428. Englewood Cliffs,
NJ: Prentice-Hall, Inc., 1980.

A reprint of a publication by the Illinois Bell Telephone Co. Medical Department. 1 figure. 19 references.

2.099 "Illinois Central Gulf Publishes Policy on Employee Alcoholism." Labor-Management Alcoholism Journal 4 (September-October 1974): 23.

Gives, in its entirety, the Illinois Central Gulf Railroad policy on employee alcoholism.

2.100 "Industry and the Troubled Employee." Alcohol Health
and Research World (Fall 1973): 12-16.

Two employee alcoholism programs (EAPs) are described
--the program at Hughes Aircraft Co. and the program at
Perfection-Cobey Co. The Hughes program began in 1967,
after a survey of programs at North American Rockwell
and other organizations. The program at Perfection-
Cobey Co., a steel-fabricating firm in Galion, Ohio,
began in 1973. 1 photograph.

2.101 "ITT Uses Alcoholism Label." Labor-Management Alcoholism Journal 4 (January-February 1975): 35-37.

The International Telephone and Telegraph (ITT) Corp.
began its employee alcoholism program (EAP) in 1973.
The program focuses on deteriorating job performance.
The program also emphasizes that alcoholism is a treatable illness, and should not be viewed as a moral problem.

2.102 Jernberg, William R. "Alcoholism Programs: Selling the
Intangible." Labor-Management Alcoholism Journal 9 (July-August 1979): 17-20.

Compares selling occupational alcoholism programs (OAPs)
to selling business life insurance. Talks about this in
terms of a market, a salesperson, and sales activity.
Market analysis, personal appearance, and the sales interview are described. Author biographical information.
1 photograph.

2.103   "Job-Induced Alcoholism and Suicide." Labour Gazette
        76 (March 1976):   125-126.

        Lawsuits against Ford Motor Co. by two former execu-
        tives and the widow of a third executive. Reasons for
        filing the lawsuits relate to occupational alcoholism.
        The lawsuits total nearly $4 million.

2.104   Jobs, Sarah Margaret. "The Effects of Alcohol on Man-
        agerial Decision-Making and Task Performance." Disser-
        tation Abstracts International 47: 1789B. Ph.D. dis-
        sertation, University of Washington, 1986. Order No.
        DA8613177.

        A simulated business game, "The Donut Fanchise," was
        central to the research for this dissertation. A major
        research instrument used was the Inhibitory Conflict
        Model.

2.105   Jones, Otto. "Kennecott's INSIGHT Program." Chapter
        in Alcoholism and Its Treatment in Industry, edited by
        Carl J. Schramm, 76-81. Baltimore, MD: Johns Hopkins
        University Press, 1977.

        INSIGHT is an employee assistance program (EAP) at the
        Utah Copper Division of Kennecott Copper Corp. The
        program, developed on July 1, 1970, refers employees,
        who have drinking problems, to appropriate treatment
        facilities in the community. This chapter looks at the
        features of the program, the goal of early identifica-
        tion, and gives an evaluation of the program.

2.106   Judd, Peter Michael. "Treatment Success in Occupation-
        al Alcoholism Programs." Dissertation Abstracts Inter-
        national 41: 2294A. Ph.D. dissertation, Brandeis Uni-
        versity, 1980. Order No. DA8024555.

        One hundred and seventy-three male alcoholics, employed
        by a private sector organization in the Detroit area,
        were the sample for this investigation. These individ-
        uals participated in the organization's occupational al-
        coholism program (OAP). The participation resulted in
        improved work performance by the employees.

2.107   Kaden, Stanley E. "Compassion or Cover-Up." The Alco-
        holic Employee." Personnel Journal 56 (July 1977):
        356-358.

        Compares two corporate employees--one blue-collar, the
        other white-collar--who are both alcoholics. Denial of
        a problem by alcoholics and others who interact with
        them is very common. Economic and other costs to in-
        dustry by worker alcoholism is huge. The success of the
        alcoholism program at Cleveland Trust Co. is discussed.
        Author biographical information.

2.108   Kane, Kevin W.   "The Corporate Responsibility in the
        Area of Alcoholism."   Personnel Journal 54 (July 1975):
        380-384.

        Alcoholic workers and their rehabilitation are described
        in terms of the economics of alcoholism, the benefits to
        employees and corporations of treatment programs, union
        participation, Alcoholics Anonymous (AA), and health in-
        surance.   The New York City Police program for alcoholic
        officers and the U.S. Government Workers program are al-
        so covered.   Author biographical information.

2.109   Karp, Robert E.   "Corporate Social Responsibility."
        Training and Development Journal 30 (November 1976):   10-
        15.

        Seven models of corporate social responsibility.   Employ-
        ee assistance program (EAP) at McDonnell Douglas Corp.,
        which was formalized in March 1970.   EAPs at: Utah Cop-
        per Division of Kennecott Copper Corp., New York City
        Transit Authority, and Caterpillar Tractor Co.   Author
        biographical information.   5 references.

2.110   Kelley, Keith P.   "The Serendipitous Dividends of an Em-
        ployee Alcoholism Program."   Labor-Management Alcoholism
        Journal 7 (September-October 1977):   39-42.

        How the employee alcoholism program (EAP) was developed
        at United California Bank (UCB).   Author biographical in-
        formation.   1 photograph.

2.111   Kemper, James S., Jr.   "Management's Role in Alcoholism
        Prevention."   Labor-Management Alcoholism Journal 7 (Jan-
        uary-February 1978):   22-23.

        Kemper Insurance and Financial Companies have contrib-
        uted to alcoholism prevention both within and outside
        the companies.   Kemper has, for example, donated funds
        to Project Teen, a Boys' Clubs of America alcoholism
        prevention program.   Kemper has also publicized in the
        Wall Street Journal, Look, and U.S. News and World Re-
        port booklets about alcohol abuse.   Author biographical
        information.   1 photograph.

2.112   "The Kemper Program: What Happens When You Have Com-
        plete Commitment from Top Management?"   Labor-Manage-
        ment Alcoholism Journal 7 (January-February 1978):   3-
        21 and 24-29.

        The Kemper Insurance and Financial Companies' Personal
        Assistance Program was set up in 1962.   This program,
        in 1977, was awarded the first National Award for the
        Most Outstanding Occupational Alcoholism Program in
        the U.S.   The award was made by the Association of La-
        bor-Management Administrators and Consultants on

Alcoholism (ALMACA).   4 photographs.   12 figures.

2.113   Kiechel, Walter, III.   "Looking Out for the Executive
Alcoholic."   _Fortune_ 105 (January 11, 1982):   117-118
and 120.

A look at executive alcoholism, including reasons why
it is difficult to easily identify who is an alcoholic.
Mentions recovered alcoholics such as insurance company
chairman, James S. Kemper, Jr. and Bruce Marsfield,
former president of Ohio Edison.   J.C. Penney and Morgan
Guaranty are two of many companies which have employee
alcoholism treatment programs.   2 illustrations.

2.114   Klingner, Donald E. and John Nalbandian.   "Case Study:
The Alcoholic Employee."   in _Public Personnel Manage-_
ment: Contexts and Strategies, by Donald E. Klingner
and John Nalbandian, 286-288.   Englewood Cliffs, NJ:
Prentice-Hall, Inc., 1985.

This case study has the dialogue of an alcoholic employee, his supervisor, and a personnel director.

2.115   Knox, A.E. Hertzler and William E. Burke.   "The Insurance Industry and Occupational Alcoholism."   _Labor Law_
Journal 26 (August 1975):   491-495.

How the Hartford Insurance Co. deals with its alcoholic
employees.   A treatment program was established in 1974.
Specific figures, regarding the economics of treatment,
are given.

2.116   Korcok, Milan.   "Alcohol on the Job--What's Being Done."
Addictions 22 (Spring 1975):   65-78.

Dominion Foundaries and Steel Corp. (DOFASCO), Ontario
Hydro, Toronto Star (newspaper), and National Steel Car
are some of the companies in Ontario concerned about,
and dealing with, the problem of alcohol on the job.
Author biographical information.   5 photographs.

2.117   Korcok, Milan.   "Alcohol on the Job--What's Being Done."
Addictions 22 (Summer 1975):   60-78.

Describes the employee assistance program (EAP) at
Douglas Aircraft Co. in Toronto.   The program is the result of joint cooperation by management, the United
Plant Guard Workers of America, and the United Auto
Workers (UAW).   Case histories of alcoholic employees
are included.   Author biographical information.   7 photographs.

2.118   Korcok, Milan.   "Alcohol on the Job--What's Being Done."
Addictions 22 (Winter 1975):   2-13.

The Lifeline Foundation is an organization which helps
small businesses--fewer than one hundred employees--deal
with alcohol abuse at work. Lloyd Fell is the director
of Lifeline. Author biographical information. 3 photographs.

2.119   Kurtz, Norman R. and Bradley Googins. "Managing the Alcoholic Employee: Towards a Model for Supervisory Intervention." Industrial Management 21 (May-June 1979):
15-21.

Planning, organizing, directing, and controlling are a
supervisor's major functions. The process for problem
intervention regarding alcoholic employees involves problem definition, identification, confrontation, referral,
and treatment. Author biographical information. 2 illustrations. 15 references.

2.120   Lambert, W.R. "Drink and Work-Discipline in Industrial
South Wales, c. 1800-1870." Welsh History Review 7
(June 1975): 289-306.

Employers, employees, and alcohol abuse in industrial
South Wales during 1800-1870. The Dowlais Iron Co.,
Pontypool Iron Works, and the Ebbw Vale Co. were three
organizations faced with alcohol-related problems. 103
footnotes.

2.121   Lawlor, Francis X. "Dupont Finds Helping Alcoholics Is
Good Business." Labor-Management Alcoholism Journal 7
(September-October 1977): 26-28.

Economics of treating alcoholic employees at E.I. Du
Pont de Nemours and Co. This treatment program dates
back to 1942. The program's success rate is about 83%.
Author biographical information. 1 photograph.

2.122   "Letter Launches New Program." Labor-Management Alcoholism Newsletter 2 (January-February 1973): 12 and 29.

Contents of a letter describing a new employee alcoholism program (EAP) at the Chicago, Milwaukee, St. Paul
and Pacific Railroad Co. The company assists its alcoholic employees through its new Office of Social Counseling. The letter was signed by C.E. Crippen, Vice
Chairman, Board of Directors.

2.123   Levens, Ernest. "The Cost-Benefit and Cost-Effective-
ness of Occupational Alcoholism Programs." Professional
Safety 21 (November 1976): 36-41.

Stresses the importance of alcoholism as a health problem and ranks it with cancer, heart disease, and mental
illness. The consequences of alcoholism are physiological, psychological, sociological, and economic in nature.

Comments on corporate alcoholism treatment programs. Du
Pont, 3M, Seaboard Coastline Railroad, Pacific Telephone
and Telegraph Co., and American Cyanamid are some of the
companies discussed. Gives the names of organizations
which provide assistance in establishing occupational alcoholism programs (OAPs): the National Council on Alcoholism (NCA), Alcoholics Anonymous (AA), the National Institute on Alcohol Abuse and Alcoholism (NIAAA), the National Clearinghouse for Alcohol Abuse Information, and
the Association of Labor and Management Administrators
and Consultants on Alcoholism (ALMACA). Abstract. 13
tables. Author biographical information. 1 photograph.
16 references.

2.124   Lindop, Stuart H.   "Three Canadian Industrial Alcoholism
Programs." Chapter in Occupational Alcoholism Programs,
edited by Richard L. Williams and Gene H. Moffat, 136-
174. Springfield, IL: Charles C. Thomas, Publisher,
1975.

Canadian industrial alcoholism programs at: Bell Canada,
Gulf Oil Canada Ltd., and Canadian National Railways
(CNR). Strengths and weaknesses of these programs are
given. 2 references.

2.125   List, Wilfred. "Helping Out the Problem Employee." Report on Business Magazine 3 (September 1986): 68-70, 72
and 76.

Employee assistance programs (EAPs) in Canada provide assistance to employees who have problems, including alcoholism. Reference is made to EAPs at companies. Warner-
Lambert Canada, Inc., CP Air, and MacMillan Bloedel are
three examples. 4 illustrations.

2.126   Lockwood, Rolf. "Dealing with the 80-Proof Employee."
Plant Management and Engineering 41 (February 1982): 20-
21.

Alcoholic employees at Stelco, Inc. in Hamilton, Ontario.
Tom Troy and Nick Siksay are Stelco staff members whose
job it is to handle this problem. Author biographical
information. 1 photograph.

2.127   Long, Richard J. "New York Bank's Program Begins with
Alcohol and Drugs, Then Grows." ABA Banking Journal 75
(September 1983): 61, 68 and 71.

The employee assistance program (EAP) at the Security
New York State Corp. in Rochester, New York is described.
Author biographical information. 2 photographs.

2.128   Lotterhos, Jerry F. "The History of Occupational Alcoholism Programming." in Occupational Alcoholism Programs, edited by Richard L. Williams and Gene H. Moffat,

26-36. Springfield, IL: Charles C. Thomas, Publisher,
1975.

Traces corporate and government efforts at dealing with
employee alcoholism from the 1940s to the 1970s. Talks
about obstacles which had to be overcome in order to
establish employee alcoholism programs (EAPs). Typical
barriers related to stereotype misconceptions about what
kind of person was an alcoholic. The skid row image of
the alcoholic was a widely held misconception. Also
gives details on how to set up an occupational alcoholism program (OAP).

2.129   Lowrey, Jane. "Sober Attitude for Tackling Alcoholism."
        Engineer 248 (February 1, 1979): 48-49.

        A comparison of how industrial alcoholism is viewed and
        dealt with in Britain and the U.S. British Rail is one
        of the relatively few British companies which have an
        alcoholism program. Nine ways of identifying an alcohol-
        ic employee are listed. 2 figures.

2.130   Luks, Allan. "Long Day's Journey into Light...How You
        Can Help the Alcoholic." Chemical Engineering 84 (May 9,
        1977): 149-150 and 152.

        Supervisors and coworkers can help alcoholic employees.
        Gives reasons why employers are hesitant to confront
        problem drinkers at work and stresses that company alco-
        holism programs are succeeding. Also states why alcohol-
        ism programs often fail. Lists eleven points which
        characterize a successful program. Gives the names of
        specific organizations which provide assistance in set-
        ting up corporate alcoholism programs. These programs
        have proven to be financially beneficial, and beneficial
        in other ways to companies, since absenteeism due to
        sickness and accidents decreases in companies which have
        the programs. Author biographical information. 1 illus-
        tration. 1 photograph.

2.131   "Lunchtime Lush Warning." Marketing 82 (October 3,
        1977): 2.

        Mac Shoub Consultants of Montreal prepared ads for the
        House of Seagram to encourage top-level executives to
        moderate their lunchtime drinking.

2.132   MacBeth, Jess and Jeffery Wiegand. "Alcoholism: A Re-
        habilitation Program That Works." Supervisory Manage-
        ment 20 (December 1975): 2-6.

        Rationale for having an employee alcoholism treatment
        program, formulating company policy regarding the pro-
        gram, implementing the program, and evaluating it. Au-
        thor biographical information. 1 illustration.

2.133   Mathis, Robert L. and John H. Jackson. "Alcoholism."
        in Personnel: Contemporary Perspectives and Applica-
        tions, by Robert L. Mathis and John H. Jackson, Sec-
        ond Edition, 396. St. Paul, MN: West Publishing Co.,
        1979.

        It is profitable for employers to establish alcohol
        rehabilitation programs for employees who have drink-
        ing problems. Some treatment success rates are as
        high as 75%. Successfully treated employees account
        for increased work productivity.

2.134   Maxwell, Ruth. "Employers." Chapter in The Booze
        Battle, by Ruth Maxwell, 135-155. New York, NY:
        Praeger Publishers, Inc., 1976.

        Industrial alcoholism programs. Examples of alcoholics
        in industry. How companies can deal effectively with
        these employees.

2.135   McCarthy, Mary-Janet. "Images of the Alcoholic Worker
        in Selected Educational Motivational Films." Disserta-
        tion Abstracts International 47: 831B. ED.D. disser-
        tation, Boston University, 1986. Order No. DA8609283.

        According to the author, industry continues to portray
        alcoholic employees in educational films as having blue-
        collar positions and low status in business environ-
        ments. This is contrary to the fact that alcoholism is
        also prevalent among white-collar workers. The author
        based her comments on an examination of seven educa-
        tional films.

2.136   McClellan, Keith. "An Overview of Occupational Alcohol-
        ism Issues for the 80's." Journal of Drug Education 12
        (1982): 1-27.

        Begins with an examination of the past decade in occu-
        pational alcoholism and employee assistance programs.
        Ends by speculating on government subsidy and the future
        EAP (employee assistance program). Earlier identifica-
        tion of employees who have a drinking problem is antici-
        pated. Essential conditions for the success of future
        programs are discussed. Author biographical information.
        Abstract. 76 references.

2.137   Megginson, Leon C. "Alcoholism." in Personnel and Hu-
        man Resources Administration, by Leon C. Megginson,
        Third Edition, 555-557. Homewood, IL: Richard D. Ir-
        win, Inc., 1977.

        Employee alcoholism as a serious problem facing person-
        nel executives.

2.138   Miethke, Richard P. "Thoughts on Evaluating an

Alcoholism Program." Journal of Occupational Medicine
18 (1976): 657.

A letter to the editor from the Medical Director, Delco
Electronics Division, General Motors (GM) Corp., Kokomo,
Indiana.

2.139   Miner, John B. and J. Frank Brewer. "Alcoholism." in
Handbook of Industrial and Organizational Psychology,
edited by Marvin D. Dunnette, 1005-1007. Chicago, IL:
Rand McNally College Publishing Co., 1976.

Overview of work and alcohol abuse.

2.140   Mondy, R. Wayne, Robert M. Noe, III and Harry N. Mills,
Jr. "Alcoholism Programs." in Personnel: The Manage-
ment of Human Resources, by R. Wayne Mondy, Robert M.
Noe, III and Harry N. Mills, Jr., 367-368. Boston, MA:
Allyn and Bacon, Inc., 1981.

Alcoholism programs in business.

2.141   Morrison, Suzanne. "Booze and Business." Toronto Board
of Trade Journal 66 (June 1976): 48-50.

Citing Addiction Research Foundation statistics, this
article claims there are over 300,000 problem drinkers
or alcoholics in Ontario. Of this number, 85% are employed. This article also talks about, in detail, an
employee assistance program (EAP) at Southam Murray, a
Toronto printing firm. The program helps employees who
have alcohol and other problems. 2 illustrations.

2.142   Murray, Robin M. "Alcoholism and Employment." Journal
of Alcoholism 10 (Spring 1975): 23-26.

The focus here is on alcoholism in the British workforce.
The relationship between occupation and alcoholism is de-
scribed. Prevention and rehabilitation are discussed.
This article is based on a lecture at the Sixth Summer
School on Alcoholism, Brighton, England, 1974. Author
biographical information. 2 tables. 21 references.

2.143   "NCA Helped Socal Change Program." Labor-Management Alcoholism Journal 7 (November-December 1977): 3-18.

Dr. Gordon W. Richmond and A.J. Sullivan are two key
people associated with establishing the employee alcoholism program (EAP) at Standard Oil of California. Sullivan is a recovered alcoholic. The program was set up in
1970. Supervisory referrals and self-referrals constitute about 95% of all referrals. 5 photographs. 6 figures.

2.144   "New Play Deals with Employed Alcoholic." Labor-Management Alcoholism Journal 6 (March-April 1977): 27.

Message in a Bottle is a play by Barbara Kay Davidson.
It deals with alcoholism in industry. Copies of the
play and/or production kits are available from either
the National Council on Alcoholism (NCA) or the Family
Service Association of America.

2.145 "Occupational Alcoholism Programs Today: Progress and
Promise." Alcohol Health and Research World (Fall
1973): 2-5.

Occupational alcoholism programs (OAPs) in the private
and public sectors, including the early beginnings of
these programs. Some of the organizations mentioned:
the National Institute on Alcohol Abuse and Alcoholism
(NIAAA), the National Council on Alcoholism (NCA), the
United Auto Workers (UAW), the Association of Labor-
Management Administrators and Consultants on Alcoholism (ALMACA), and the Yale Center of Alcohol Studies.
4 illustrations.

2.146 Olcott, William A. "Alcoholism: Managers Can Now Do
More Than Just Wring Their Hands." Office Administration and Automation 45 (November 1984): 9.

Misconceptions, stereotypes, and stigma regarding alcoholism, and what managers can do about this. 1 photograph.

2.147 Olkinuora, Martti. "Alcoholism and Occupation." Scan-
dinavian Journal of Work, Environment and Health 10
(1984): 511-515.

Alcoholism and occupation with an emphasis on Finland.
Mortality statistics for death from cirrhosis of the
liver, use of health services for alcoholism, and risk
factors for alcohol-related problems in occupations are
analyzed. Author biographical information. Abstract.
8 tables. 14 references.

2.148 Orr, Michael. "Business and the Compulsive Drinker."
Addictions 38 (Summer 1972): 38-43.

The importance to Canadian employers and employees of
detecting alcoholism early. Kodak Canada, the Royal
Bank, Imperial Oil, and Bell Canada are examples of
companies in Canada which have employee alcoholism programs (EAPs). The Bell Canada program was established
in 1951. The May Street Centre, an Addiction Research
Foundation clinic in Toronto, provides treatment for
employed alcoholics. 1 illustration.

2.149 Pati, Gopal C. and John I. Adkins, Jr. "The Employer's
Role in Alcoholism Assistance." Personnel Journal 62
(July 1983): 568-572.

Major features of this article: statistics on the
characteristics of alcoholics, assistance for smaller
companies, identifying and counseling the problem employee, and a supervisor's checklist. Author biographical information. 2 figures. 6 references.

2.150   "Penney Produces Training Film." Labor-Management Alcoholism Journal 7 (January-February 1978): 32-33.

"Here's Looking at You" is a twenty-eight-minute color
film about job performance and alcoholism. The J.C.
Penney Co. produced the film. 1 photograph.

2.151   Perham, John. "Battling Employee Alcoholism." Dun's
Business Month 119 (June 1982): 48-49 and 53.

Between 1973 and 1982, according to a survey by Dun's
Business Month, the number of U.S. companies with alco-
holism programs increased from 400 to more than 5,000.
Examples of companies with these programs: Mobil Corp.,
Xerox, United Airlines, Union Pacific Railroad, and
United Technologies Corp. 1 photograph.

2.152   Perkins, George. "Alcoholism in the Workplace." Management World 7 (February 1978): 6-8 and 10.

Views alcoholism as a major physical, mental health,
and social problem. Sees alcoholism as an economic liability to society. Elaborates on ways to treat alcoholism: physical illness treatment, legal intervention,
family intervention, and job intervention. Lists ten
criteria for an effective occupational intervention program. Author biographical information.

2.153   Peterson, Richard B. and Lane Tracy. "Alcoholism." in
Systematic Management of Human Resources, by Richard B.
Peterson and Lane Tracy, 250-251. Reading, MA: Addi-
son-Wesley Publishing Co., 1979.

How management should deal with alcoholic employees.

2.154   Phillips, Donald A. and Patricia Allen. "Meet Sally and
Jim, Successful Bank Execs--and Recovering Alcoholics."
ABA Banking Journal 75 (September 1983): 61-62 and 67.

The First Interstate Bank of California, the National
City Bank of Cleveland, and Morgan Guaranty Trust Co. of
New York all have employee alcoholism programs (EAPs).
The cost of the National City Bank of Cleveland program
is $60,000.00 annually. This program saves the bank
$800,000.00 each year. Author biographical information.
2 photographs.

2.155   Phillips, Donald A. and Harry J. Older. "Alcoholic Employees Beget Troubled Supervisors." Supervisory

Management 26 (September 1981): 2-9.

Anger, guilt, fear, and denial are feelings supervisors
are likely to experience in their work with alcoholic
employees. Effective supervisory action is also hinder-
ed by management barriers such as long-felt prejudices
and fears. Supervisors, in view of this, sometimes require counseling. Author biographical information. 1
illustration.

2.156 Pike, Thomas P. "Alcoholism in the Executive Suite."
       Vital Speeches of the Day 46 (January 1, 1980): 166-
       169.

       Text of a speech about an alcoholic executive. The
       speaker is Thomas P. Pike, Honorary Vice Chairman of the
       Board, Fluor Corp. Pike used to be an alcoholic. Au-
       thor biographical information.

2.157 "Pioneer Program Honored." Labor-Management Alcoholism
       Newsletter 2 (July-August 1972): 17-21.

       A look, thirty years later, at the employee alcoholism
       program (EAP) at E.I. du Pont de Nemours and Co. The
       company's medical director received, on the occasion of
       the program's thirtieth anniversary, a congratulatory
       letter from President Richard Nixon.

2.158 Poe, Randall. "Lost Weeks." Across the Board 17 (Ju-
       ly 1980): 70.

       Reviews a Conference Board study about alcoholism in
       American industry. The study is by Richard M. Weiss.
       More than 1300 corporations were surveyed for the study.
       More than 75% of corporate alcoholism treatment programs
       were established in 1970 or later. 1 cartoon illustra-
       tion.

2.159 Poley, Wayne, Gary Lea and Gail Vibe. "Company Poli-
       cies." in Alcoholism: A Treatment Manual, by Wayne
       Poley, Gary Lea and Gail Vibe, 57-58. New York, NY:
       Gardner Press, Inc., 1979.

       Example of an employer policy on alcohol and drug abuse.

2.160 Poley, Wayne, Gary Lea and Gail Vibe. "Identification
       of the Alcoholic Employee." in Alcoholism: A Treatment
       Manual, by Wayne Poley, Gary Lea and Gail Vibe, 55. New
       York, NY: Gardner Press, Inc., 1979.

       Six things for the supervisor to bear in mind in iden-
       tifying the alcoholic employee: poor work performance,
       absenteeism, physical appearance, poor health, safety,
       and poor work relations.

2.161   Poley, Wayne, Gary Lea and Gail Vibe. "Industrial Al-
         coholism Programs." in <u>Alcoholism: A Treatment Manu-</u>
         <u>al</u>, by Wayne Poley, Gary Lea and Gail Vibe, 52-54.
         New York, NY: Gardner Press, Inc., 1979.

         Facts and figures about alcoholism in industry. De-
         scribes occupational alcoholism programs (OAPs).

2.162   Poley, Wayne, Gary Lea and Gail Vibe. "Interviewing
         Procedures." in <u>Alcoholism: A Treatment Manual</u>, by
         Wayne Poley, Gary Lea and Gail Vibe, 55-56. New York,
         NY: Gardner Press, Inc., 1979.

         Nine steps to follow in interviewing the alcoholic em-
         ployee: prepare a written fact sheet, keep discussion
         on the subject, offer assistance, be optimistic, avoid
         meaningless threats, never cover up, do not diagnose,
         do not betray confidence, and close the interview.

2.163   Poley, Wayne, Gary Lea and Gail Vibe. "Job-Based
         Risks." in <u>Alcoholism: A Treatment Manual</u>, by Wayne
         Poley, Gary Lea and Gail Vibe, 58. New York, NY:
         Gardner Press, Inc., 1979.

         Outlines four categories of factors related to work
         which increase the likelihood of employee alcoholism.

2.164   Poley, Wayne, Gary Lea and Gail Vibe. "Referral Proce-
         dure." in <u>Alcoholism: A Treatment Manual</u>, by Wayne
         Poley, Gary Lea and Gail Vibe, 56-57. New York, NY:
         Gardner Press, Inc., 1979.

         Referring the alcoholic employee for treatment. What to
         do about employees who do not cooperate, that is, admit
         they have a problem.

2.165   Poley, Wayne, Gary Lea and Gail Vibe. "Role of the Su-
         pervisor." in <u>Alcoholism: A Treatment Manual</u>, by Wayne
         Poley, Gary Lea and Gail Vibe, 54. New York, NY: Gard-
         ner Press, Inc., 1979.

         Crucial role of the supervisor in identifying the alco-
         holic employee.

2.166   "Project Finds Jobs for Recovering Alcoholics." <u>Labor-</u>
         <u>Management Alcoholism Journal</u> 6 (January-February 1977):
         38.

         The Union Carbide Corp. provided a grant to the National
         Council on Alcoholism (NCA) to help recovering alcohol-
         ics find jobs in the New York area. The person in charge
         of the program is Bud Laupheimer.

2.167   Ralston, August. "Employee Alcoholism: Responses of the
         Largest Industrials." <u>Personnel Administrator</u> 22

August 1977):   50-52 and 54-56.

Reports on a questionnaire survey of fifty U.S. industrial corporations, regarding alcoholic employee rehabilitation programs. Thirty-five (70%) of the corporations surveyed responded. The corporations were ranked
by asset size in Fortune magazine. Author biographical
information. 3 tables. 16 references.

2.168   Ravin, Iver S. "Formulation of an Alcoholism Rehabili-
        tation Program at Boston Edison Company." Chapter in
        Occupational Alcoholism Programs, edited by Richard L.
        Williams and Gene H. Moffat, 194-223. Springfield, IL:
        Charles C. Thomas, Publisher, 1975.

        An alcoholism rehabilitation program was set up in 1963
        at Boston Edison Co. When the program was evaluated in
        1973, a significant finding was that the program had a
        77% recovery rate. The program was also found to be
        cost effective. 5 tables. 2 appendices.

2.169   Reiman, Tyrus. "Companies and Unions Cooperate to Fight
        Alcoholism." Canadian Mining Journal 104 (June 1983):
        21-22.

        Employee assistance programs (EAPs) at mining companies
        in Canada, including Hudson Bay Mining and Smelting,
        Cullaton Lake Gold Mines, and Sherritt Gordon. 1 photo-
        graph.

2.170   Reiman, Tyrus. "The Rise of the EAP." Benefits Canada
        7 (July-August 1983): 18-20.

        The employee assistance program (EAP) provides aid to
        company employees who have a variety of personal prob-
        lems, for example, alcoholism. Comments on EAPs at
        Canadian companies: Imperial Oil Ltd., Falconbridge,
        MacMillan Bloedel Ltd., CN Rail, and Shell Canada. Men-
        tions INPUT'83, the Fifth Biennial Canadian Conference
        scheduled for August 9-12, 1983 at the Sheraton Centre
        in Toronto. EAPs are to be discussed at INPUT '83. 2
        illustrations. Author biographical information.

2.171   Reynolds, Barbara. "How Industry Can Help the Alcohol-
        ic." Human Needs 1 (February 1973): 5-8.

        Describes an industry-oriented alcoholism program in
        Milwaukee, Wisconsin. The program is sponsored by the
        DePaul Rehabilitation Hospital and the Wisconsin Divi-
        sion of Vocational Rehabilitation (DVR). The DePaul
        Sertoma Simulated Workshop also provides assistance to
        alcoholics. 8 photographs.

2.172   Rich, Philip. "Dealing with Alcoholism in U.S. Indus-
        try." USA Today 109 (July 1980): 26-29.

The first company in the U.S. to establish an alcoholism
treatment program for its staff was Du Pont in 1943.
This article also mentions the recovery rate for employee alcoholism treatment programs at Illinois Bell Telephone Co., Eastman Kodak, and Minnesota Mining and Manufacturing. There are twelve points to use as a guide
in implementing an occupational alcoholism program
(OAP). Also covered is what chracterizes an ineffective
OAP. Author biographical information. 1 sketch. 7
notes.

2.173   "R.J. Reynolds: An Unusual Success Story." Labor-Man-
        agement Alcoholism Newsletter 2 (March-April 1973): 1-
        14.

        The employee alcoholism program (EAP) at the R.J. Reyn-
        olds Tobacco Co. in Winston-Salem, North Carolina. This
        article has an excerpt from the personnel policy and
        procedure manual entitled; "Program for Employees with
        Drinking Problems." 3 photographs. 3 figures.

2.174   Roberts, James S. "Drink and Industrial Work Discipline
        in 19th Century Germany." Journal of Social History 15
        (Fall 1981): 25-38.

        Based on research for the author's 1979 doctoral dis-
        sertation at the University of Iowa, Drink, Temperance
        and the Working Class in 19th Century Germany. Author
        biographical information. 60 footnotes.

2.175   Roche, James M. "Alcoholism: The Disease in Industry."
        Vital Speeches of the Day 39 (December 1, 1972): 120-
        121.

        Remarks of James M. Roche, former chairman of the board,
        General Motors Corp., delivered before the Alcoholism
        Foundation, New York, October 3, 1972. Roche spoke
        about the General Motors (GM) employee alcoholism reha-
        bilitation program. Author biographical information.

2.176   Roman, Paul. M. Barriers to the Use of Constructive Con-
        frontation with Employed Alcoholics." Journal of Drug
        Issues 12 (1982): 369-382.

        There are four barriers to the use of constructive con-
        frontation with employed alcoholics: organizational
        management ideologies, the value orientations of Amer-
        ican society, the medicalization of employee perfor-
        mance problems, and the professionalization of means for
        handling these problems. Author biographical information
        Abstract. 26 references.

2.177   Roman, Paul M. "Employee Assistance Programs in Austra-
        lia and the United States: Comparisons of Origin,
        Structure, and the Role of Behavioral Science Research."

Journal of Applied Behavioral Science 19 (1983): 367-379.

Industrial alcoholism programs in the U.S. in the 1940s were precursors to employee assistance programs (EAPs). The author spent four weeks in Australia carrying out research for this article. Author biographical information. 1 note. 2 reference notes. 24 references.

2.178   Roman, Paul M. "From Employee Alcoholism to Employee Assistance: Deemphases on Prevention and Alcohol Problems in Work-Based Programs." *Journal of Studies on Alcohol* 42 (1981): 244-272.

Transition from employee alcoholism to employee assistance programs (EAPs), and the change in emphasis from prevention and constructive confrontation to self-referrals for counseling and treatment. Abstract. Author biographical information. 5 footnotes. 68 references.

2.179   Roseman, Edward. "The Alcoholic Employee." Chapter in *Managing the Problem Employee*, by Edward Roseman, 191-196. New York, NY: American Management Associations, 1982.

Uses case histories and dialogue to illustrate how managers should deal with alcoholic employees.

2.180   Royal College of Psychiatrists. "Drinking Problems and Employment." in *Alcohol and Alcoholism: The Report of a Special Committee of the Royal College of Psychiatrists*, by Royal College of Psychiatrists, 62-63. London: Tavistock Publications Ltd., 1979.

A drinking problem results in other problems for the alcoholic employee. Even if he is not dismissed, and is not treated for his alcoholism, he may have to retire early or may be promoted laterally.

2.181   Royce, James E. "Occupational Programs." Chapter in *Alcohol Problems and Alcoholism: A Comprehensive Survey*, by James E. Royce, 197-210. New York, NY: Free Press, 1981.

Explains why occupational alcoholism programs (OAPs) in industry and government are successful. Contends that these programs help employers save money. Stresses the importance of confidentiality between the alcoholic employee and the alcoholism counselor. Also stresses the importance of family involvement in the rehabilitation process. 15 references.

2.182   Rutherford, Derek. "Alcoholic Solution." *Accountant* 183 (August 21, 1980): 309-310.

Relationship between executives, stress, and excessive drinking. A list of twenty-six questions helps evaluate the extent of a person's alcohol consumption. Author biographical information. 1 chart.

2.183   Sager, Leon B. "The Corporation and the Alcoholic." Across the Board 16 (June 1979): 79-82.

Allis Chalmers, Consolidated Edison, Great Northern Railway, Detroit Edison, Du Pont, Minnesota Mining, and People's Light and Coke Co. all report varying degrees of success with their employee alcoholism programs (EAPs). Author biographical information. 1 cartoon illustration.

2.184   Sager, Leon B. "Our Ten Million Problem Drinkers: What's Being Done About It." CLU Journal 32 (October 1978): 38-46.

After discussing successful alcoholism treatment programs in corporations, this article looks at other organizations which fight alcoholism. Three latter organizations are: Alcoholics Anonymous (AA), the Johnston Institute (Minneapolis, Minnesota) and the Menninger Foundation (Topeka, Kansas). A table lists twenty-eight organizations in relation to: number of employees, number of programs, number of years, cost, estimated savings, and percent recovery rate. Author biographical information. 10 footnotes. 1 table.

2.185   Salazar, Leo and Robert Doyle. "The Alcoholism Program at the Bethlehem Steel Company: The Importance of Supervisory Training." Maryland State Medical Journal 27 (July 1978): 80-81.

The role of supervisors at Bethlehem Steel is vital to the success of that company's industrial alcoholism program. Alcoholism workshops were held for supervisors in August 1977 at Bethlehem's plant in Sparrow's Point, Maryland. The workshops helped increase referrals to the alcoholism program. Author biographical information.

2.186   Sammons, Donna. "Alcoholism in the Workplace." Chemical Engineering 86 (August 27, 1979): 109-110.

Twenty-five questions developed by the National Council on Alcoholism (NCA) help a person know if he is becoming an alcoholic. The latter part of this article is about the effect of alcohol on employee work habits. Author biographical information.

2.187   "Sandia Laboratories Announces Alcoholism Policy." Labor-Management Alcoholism Newsletter 2 (November-December 1972): 18-20.

Employee alcoholism policy of Sandia Laboratories of
Albuquerque, New Mexico. Other Sandia facilities are
located in Livermore, California and Tonopah, Nevada.

2.188   Sanzotta, Donald.   "Alcoholism on the Job." in The
        Manager's Guide to Interpersonal Relations, by Donald
        Sanzotta, 151-153. New York, NY: AMACOM, 1979.

        Problem drinkers cost industry $10 billion annually.
        Managers should realize that staff personal problems,
        involving alcohol, can become organizational problems.
        When this occurs, managers must know how to handle al-
        coholic employees.

2.189   Schaeffer, Dorothy.   "Alcoholism: Challenge for To-
        day's Supervisor." Supervision 41 (September 1979):
        11-13.

        How supervisors can recognize the stages of alcoholism
        and the proper way for supervisors to deal with, and
        assist, alcoholic employees. 1 photograph.

2.190   Schramm, Carl J.   "Evaluating Industrial Alcoholism
        Programs: A Human-Capital Approach." Journal of Studies
        on Alcohol 41 (1980): 702-713.

        The author proposes that a human-capital model can be
        used to explain why businesses decide to set up, or to
        continue established, employee alcoholism treatment pro-
        grams. He reviews nine evaluative studies and discusses
        human-capital theory. This theory views employees as
        investments, just as machinery and inventory are seen as
        investments. A positive return on investment is expect-
        ed when an employer deals positively with his employees.
        Providing employees with safe working conditions and
        health care are two ways to invest in staff. Author
        biographical information. Abstract. 1 table. 1 fig-
        ure. 28 references.

2.191   Schramm, Carl J. and Robert J. DeFillippi.   "Character-
        istics of Successful Alcoholism Treatment Programs for
        American Workers." British Journal of Addiction 70
        (1975): 271-275.

        Research by the authors included an evaluation of twen-
        ty-four previous studies, concerning successful indus-
        trial alcoholism treatment programs. The authors also
        examined the effect of company coercion and confronta-
        tion on the successful identification and referral of
        alcoholic employees. Author biographical information.
        Abstract. 24 references.

2.192   Sherman, Paul A.   "The Alcoholic Executive." Chapter
        in Occupational Clinical Psychology, edited by James
        S.J. Manuso, 45-54. New York, NY: Praeger Publishers,

1983.

History of occupational programs, beginning with the
1930s. Describes what constitutes an occupational program. Followed by a look at executive alcoholism, including successful intervention and treatment of the
executive alcoholic. 26 references.

2.193   Shirley, Donald. "What Does It Take to 'Sell' an Ef-
        fective Program?" Labor-Management Alcoholism Journal
        6 (September-October 1976): 22-23.

        Effectively communicating with the chief executive offi-
        cer (CEO) of a company is essential if an employee alco-
        holism program (EAP) is to be effective. Eight key el-
        ments in a EAP are listed. Four reasons are given why
        a program may be ineffective. Three ways to present the
        program to a CEO are outlined. Author biographical in-
        formation. 1 photograph.

2.194   Sikula, Andrew F. and John F. McKenna. "Alcoholsm."
        in The Management of Human Resources: Personnel Text
        and Current Issues, by Andrew F. Sikula and John F. Mc-
        Kenna, 328. New York, NY: John Wiley and Sons, 1984.

        The value to employees and employers of employee alco-
        holism programs (EAPs) is illustrated with the example
        of General Motors (GM).

2.195   Silburt, David. "Substance Abuse: The Monster That
        Hides in the Dark." Occupational Health and Safety
        Canada 2 (November-December 1986): 26-30 and 59.

        Employee alcohol and drug abuse in Canadian industry.
        Employee assistance programs (EAPs). Representatives
        from the Addiction Research Foundation (ARF), Canadian
        Auto Workers, Alberta Alcoholism and Drug Abuse Com-
        mission (AADAC), and the Donwood Institute comment.
        Author biographical information. 3 photographs.

2.196   Sinclair, Sonja. "Alcoholism Is Industry's Business."
        Canadian Business 45 (November 1972): 10-12.

        Alcoholism in Canadian industry. Statistics about alco-
        holic employees. Discusses constructive coercion, a
        strategy used by companies to compel problem drinkers
        to seek help. Dofasco, Canadian National Railways (CNR),
        and General Motors (GM) Canada are three Canadian com-
        panies which have alcoholism treatment programs for al-
        coholic employees. 1 photograph.

2.197   Sinclair, Sonja. "How Three Employers Fight Addiction
        Problems." Canadian Business 45 (November 1972): 14-
        16.

There are five vital elements in successful alcoholism treatment programs: a statement of company policy, identification of the alcoholic employee, confrontation with the employee, diagnosis and referral, and treatment and follow-up. Ontario Hydro, Dofasco, and the Ontario government endorse these elements. 3 photographs.

2.198   Singbeil, Beverly. "Bottle Tactics: The Corporate War against Alcoholism." Business Life (February-March 1983): 35-38.

Focuses on employee alcoholism and employer alcoholism treatment programs in Canada. Comments on the employee assistance programs (EAPs) of Canadian National Railways (CNR), Gulf Canada Ltd., MacMillan Bloedel, and the Royal Bank. 2 sketches.

2.199   Smith, Archibald Ian. "The Effects of Alcohol on Aspects of Business Decision-Making." Dissertation Abstracts International 41: 4690B-4691B. Ph.D. dissertation, University of Western Ontario, 1980.

In this research, concerning the effects of alcohol on aspects of business decision-making behavior, independent experiments took into account variables such as task risk, alcohol dose, social drinking history, and need for achievement. The expected value (EV) model and the Atkinson model of decision-making were also used.

2.200   Smith, Jackson. "Alcoholism: Addiction and Affliction." Chapter in Drug Abuse in Industry: Growing Corporate Dilemma, edited by Jordan M. Scher, 221-227. Springfield, IL: Charles C. Thomas, 1973.

Overview of alcoholism.

2.201   Smith, Robert. "Confessions of an Alcoholic Executive." Dun's 99 (June 1972): 72-74 and 79.

A first-person account by an advertising and marketing executive about his alcoholism. 1 photograph.

2.202   Smithers, R. Brinkley. "Alcoholism Program Administration: Measures of Effectiveness." Labor-Management Alcoholism Journal 6 (January-February 1977): 20-21.

Facts and figures about the General Motors (GM) Corp. employee alcoholism program (EAP) illustrate alcoholism program administration effectiveness. Author biographical information. 1 photograph.

2.203   Sullivan, Roger M., Jr. "Balancing the Rights of the Alcoholic Employee with the Legitimate Concerns of the Employer: Reasonable Accommodation Vs Undue Hardship."

Montana Law Review 46 (Summer 1985):   401-418.

Employment discrimination claims by alcoholic employees under federal law and Montana law are the two main topics dealt with in this article. 100 footnotes.

2.204   Surles, Carol Diann Smith. "Historical Development of Alcoholism Control Programs in Industry from 1940-1978." Dissertation Abstracts International 39: 5995A. Ph.D. dissertation, University of Michigan, 1978.

The author used historical research techniques and obtained primary and secondary evidence. She discusses a number of influences in the development of industrial alcoholism control programs. Five influences: Alcoholics Anonymous (AA), American Medical Association (AMA), Rutgers Center of Alcohol Studies, federal involvement, and labor unions.

2.205   Tapscott, John. "The Des Moines Success Story: How a Council Organized Many Local Companies as Participants in a Cooperative Employee Alcoholism Program." Labor-Management Alcoholism Journal 8 (July-August 1978):   25-31.

Some of the employer organizations with which the National Council on Alcoholism (NCA) has employee alcoholism programs (EAPs) in effect: Continental Western Insurance Co., Dial Financial Corp., Airline Textile Manufacturing Co., Iowa-Des Moines National Bank, Central Life Assurance Co., American Federal Savings, Pittsburgh Des Moines Steel, Super Valu Stores, Inc., and the Hiland Potato Chip Co. Author biographical information. 1 photograph. 3 figures.

2.206   Tavernier, Gerard. "Corporate Aid for the Alcoholic." International Management 34 (July 1979):   16-20.

Corporate alcoholism programs in a number of countries, including the U.S., Britain, France, and West Germany. A few of the companies are: Caterpillar Tractor Co. and Pacific Telephone and Telegraph Co. (United Sates), Regie Nationale des Usines Renault (France), and Bayer AG, Thyssen Niederrhein AG, Peine-Salzgitter AG, and BASF AG (West Germany). An inset section is entitled "Alcoholism and the Executive." 3 photographs.

2.207   Tersine, Richard J. and James Hazeldine. "Alcoholism: A Productivity Hangover." Business Horizons 25 (November-December 1982): 68-72.

This article consists of four main parts: the measurement of productivity loss, job performance, legal issues, and employee assistance programs (EAPs). Lists fifteen characteristics common to most alcoholics.

Mentions employee alcoholism treatment programs at Du Pont, Eastman Kodak, General Motors (GM), Firestone, and the Great Northern Railway Co. Author biographical information. 13 footnotes.

2.208   Thomas, Lisa A. and Paul M. Roman. "A Factor Analytic Study of Emerging Work Styles among Occupational Alcoholism Program Consultants." Journal of Drug Issues 11 (1981): 293-310.

An examination, in terms of work styles, of occupational alcoholism consultants at state and local levels. This occupation arose in the early 1970s. Data for this study was obtained from 306 of these consultants. Author biographical information. Abstract. 7 tables. 18 references.

2.209   Travers, Denis J. "Policies in Australia." Chapter in Alcohol Problems in Employment, edited by Brian D. Hore and Martin A. Plant, 185-195. London: Croom Helm Ltd., 1981.

In 1972 in Australia there was only one company with a policy regarding employee alcoholism--Kodak Australasia Pty. Ltd. Six years later the number of employee alcoholism programs (EAPs) in industry and government was 127.

2.210   Trice, Harrison M. and Janice M. Beyer. "A Data-Based Examination of Selection-Bias in the Evaluation of a Job-Based Alcoholism Program." Alcoholism: Clinical and Experimental Research 5 (Fall 1981): 489-496.

Describes constructive confrontation, a strategy used to convince alcoholic employees to seek treatment for alcoholism. A major source of data used in this study consisted of employee records for employees being treated for drinking problems. The data covered the years 1964-1977. The employees worked for a large national corporation. Supervisors who supervised two types of problem employees were interviewed--those who dealt with alcoholic employees, and those who dealt with employees who had nonalcoholic problems. This paper was presented at the Annual Medical-Scientific Meeting, National Council on Alcoholism (NCA), Seattle, Washington, May 1980. Abstract. Author biographical information. 36 references.

2.211   Trice, Harrison M. and Janice M. Beyer. "Work-Related Outcomes of the Constructive-Confrontation Strategy in a Job-Based Alcoholism Program." Journal of Studies on Alcohol 45 (1984): 393-404.

This study investigated how supervisors dealt with two types of problem employees--problem drinkers and

employees with other problems. Over 600 managers in a
major U.S. corporation were interviewed. The supervisors of problem drinkers took more action in dealing
with these individuals than did the supervisors of problem employees who did not have a drinking problem. Author biographical information. Abstract. 5 tables.
35 references.

2.212   Trice, Harrison M. and Paul M. Roman. "Absenteeism:
        Impact of Deviant Drinking." in Spirits and Demons at
        Work: Alcohol and Other Drugs on the Job, by Harrison
        M. Trice and Paul M. Roman, Second Edition, 134-138.
        Ithaca, NY: New York State School of Industrial and
        Labor Relations Cornell University, 1978.

        Compares work absenteeism of high-status deviant drink-
        ers and low-status deviant drinkers.

2.213   Trice, Harrison M. and Paul M. Roman. "The Costs of De-
        viant Drinking to the Employer." in Spirits and Demons
        at Work: Alcohol and Other Drugs on the Job, by Harri-
        son M. Trice and Paul M. Roman, Second Edition, 2-9.
        Ithaca, NY: New York State School of Industrial and
        Labor Relations Cornell University, 1978.

        The costs of deviant drinking to the employer are not
        only economic costs reflected in inefficiency on the
        job and in employee absenteeism. Interpersonal fric-
        tion--especially that associated with problem drinkers
        and their supervisors--reflects a non-economic cost.

2.214   Trice, Harrison M. and Paul M. Roman. "Cover-Up: The
        Deviant Drinker." in Spirits and Demons at Work: Al-
        cohol and Other Drugs on the Job, by Harrison M. Trice
        and Paul M. Roman, Second Edition, 132-133. Ithaca,
        NY: New York State School of Industrial and Labor Re-
        lations Cornell University, 1978.

        How deviant drinkers cover up their job-related drink-
        ing. How work associates help deviant drinkers conceal
        their drinking.

2.215   Trice, Harrison M. and Paul M. Roman. "Turnover: Im-
        pact of Deviant Drinking." in Spirits and Demons at
        Work: Alcohol and Other Drugs on the Job, by Harrison
        M. Trice and Paul M. Roman, Second Edition, 130. Itha-
        ca, NY: New York State School of Industrial and Labor
        Relations Cornell University, 1978.

        Contrary to stereotypes, deviant-drinking employees do
        not change jobs frequently. These individuals are not
        "job hoppers."

2.216   Trice, Harrison M. and Paul M. Roman. "Work Efficiency:
        Impact of Deviant Drinking." in Spirits and Demons at

Work: Alcohol and Other Drugs on the Job, by Harrison
M. Trice and Paul M. Roman, Second Edition, 125-126.
Ithaca, NY: New York State School of Industrial and
Labor Relations Cornell University, 1978.

Reference is made to studies which associate deviant
drinking with declining work performance, including two
studies by Alcoholics Anonymous (AA).

2.217   Trice, Harrison M. and Mona Schonbrunn. "A History of
Job-Based Alcoholism Programs: 1900-1955." Journal
of Drug Issues 11 (1981): 171-198.

Two of the most important influences in the history of
job-based alcoholism programs were World War II--its
impact on the labor market--and Alcoholics Anonymous
(AA). Author biographical information. Abstract. 51
references.

2.218   "Troubled Employee." Association Management 35 (March
1983): 71 and 73.

Ten early-warning signs of occupational alcoholism,
provided by the American Association of Medical Society
Executives. Poor job performance as rationale for confronting alcoholic employees. Denial by these employees of a drinking problem. Role of consultants in identifying corporate alcoholics. 1 illustration.

2.219   "'Troubled Employees' Rehabilitation Seen Profitable to
Business." National Underwriter: Life and Health Insurance Edition 81 (November 12, 1977): 17.

It is more profitable to a company to rehabilitate alcoholic employees than it is to terminate them. Two people addressing a meeting in Toronto, of the Association
of Life Insurance Medical Directors of America, made
this claim. A.E. Hertzler Knox (Hartford Group) and
Samuel B. Harper (Cuna Mutual) were the speakers. The
Hartford Group has a computer program which demonstrates
the cost-benefit ratio of the company's guidance program.

2.220   "Union Pacific on the Right Track." Labor-Management
Alcoholism Newsletter 2 (January-February 1973): 11-12.

Text of a letter by J.C. Kenefick, President, Union Pacific Railroad Co. The letter, distributed to all employees, discusses the Union Pacific employee alcoholism
program (EAP). The letter was incorporated into a six-
page leaflet which describes the alcoholism program.

2.221   "UP Is a Good Direction." Labor-Management Alcoholism
Journal 4 (September-October 1974): 1-16.

The Union Pacific Railroad Co. launched its employee assistance program (EAP) on December 1, 1972. 5 photographs. 5 figures.

2.222   von Wiegand, Ross A. "Alcoholism in Industry (U.S.A.)."
British Journal of Addiction 67 (1972): 181-187.

U.S. Steel, Goodyear Rubber, Kennecott Copper, United
Bank of California, and the Kemper Insurance Co. are
among the U.S. companies which have employee alcoholism
programs (EAPs). There is union support for such programs from the Teamsters, United Auto Workers (UAW), and
other unions. In government, the United States Civil
Service Commission is developing an employee alcoholism
program. In 1972, an estimated 300 U.S. companies had
this type of program. Author biographical information.
Abstract.

2.223   von, Wiegand, Ross A. "Don't Look for Alcoholics!" Labor-Management Alcoholism Newsletter 2 (July-August
1972):   14-15.

The way to effectively deal with employee alcoholism is
to focus on job performance--not look for employees who
are alcoholics.

2.224   Walker, Joseph J. "Supervising the Alcoholic." Supervisory Management 23 (November 1978): 26-32.

Nine supervisory guidelines to follow in supervising
the alcoholic worker. An inset section is entitled
"Supervisors' Do's and Don'ts: How to Handle a Troubled
Employee." This section lists ten points. Author biographical information. 1 illustration.

2.225   Walsh, Diana Chapman and Ralph W. Hingson. "Where to
Refer Employees for Treatment of Drinking Problems: The
Limited Lessons from Empirical Research." Journal of
Occupational Medicine 27 (1985): 745-752.

The need for clearer definitions of terms is required in
discussing occupational alcoholism programs (OAPs), as
is data about the effectiveness of these programs. The
assessment and referral process is another area that requires further study. Author biographical information.
Abstract. 71 references.

2.226   Weiner, Jack B. "On the Job: Industry's $15 Billion
Hangover." Chapter in Drinking, by Jack B. Weiner, 40-
56. New York, NY: W.W. Norton and Co., Inc., 1976.

Reports on employee alcoholism programs (EAPs) in industry. A few of the companies covered include: Firestone Tire and Rubber, United California Bank, Hughes

Aircraft, and General Motors (GM).

2.227   Weiss, Richard M.   "Company Practices."   Chapter in
        Dealing with Alcoholism in the Workplace, by Richard M.
        Weiss, 9-13.   New York, NY: Conference Board, Inc.,
        1980.

        Examples of company responses to employee alcoholism.
        A high technology manufacturer, a farm equipment com-
        pany, a paper goods manufacturer, a publishing company,
        a mineral company, and an aerospace manufacturer are
        companies mentioned.   2 tables.

2.228   Weiss, Richard M.   "Determining the Effects of Alcohol
        Abuse on Employee Productivity."   American Psychologist
        40 (May 1985):   578-580.

        Questions the evidence used in studies about the nega-
        tive effect of alcohol abuse on employee productivity.
        Author biographical information.   23 references.

2.229   Weiss, Richard M.   "The Effects of Occupational Pro-
        grams."   Chapter in Dealing with Alcoholism in the Work-
        place, by Richard M. Weiss, 28-40.   New York, NY: Con-
        ference Board, Inc., 1980.

        Drinking behavior and job status are two variables dis-
        cussed in relation to the effects of occupational alco-
        holism programs (OAPs).   A comparison is made between
        employees who referred themselves into the treatment
        program, and employees who were referred into the pro-
        gram by supervisors.   7 exhibits.   1 table.

2.230   Weiss, Richard M.   "Executive Attitudes, Perceptions
        and Programs."   Chapter in Dealing with Alcoholism in
        the Workplace, by Richard M. Weiss, 4-8.   New York, NY:
        Conference Board, Inc., 1980.

        Executive attitudes about: alcoholism treatment, per-
        ceptions of the causes of alcoholism, and perceptions
        about program implementation and results.   7 tables.   1
        chart.

2.231   Weiss, Richard M.   "Gaining Employee Acceptance."   Chap-
        ter in Dealing with Alcoholism in the Workplace, by
        Richard M. Weiss, 19-27.   New York, NY: Conference
        Board, Inc., 1980.

        Emphasis on: techniques used for disseminating informa-
        tion about corporate alcoholism programs, training and
        educational sessions, training program staff, diagnosing
        alcoholism, referral for treatment, and program access
        for employees' dependents.   3 tables.   5 charts.

2.232   Weiss, Richard M.   "The Supervisor's Role."   Chapter in

Dealing with Alcoholism in the Workplace, by Richard M. Weiss, 14-18. New York, NY: Conference Board, Inc., 1980.

Role of supervisors in dealing with alcoholic employees in a number of work environments: chemical, public utility, farm equipment, insurance, bank, consumer products, laboratory, and telephone. 1 table.

2.233   Welty, Gus. "Don't Fire Him--Help Him." Railway Age 174 (June 25, 1973): 16.

Employee alcoholism in a railway context at Great Northern and Burlington Northern. Safety performance, company/union relationships, and family life benefit from staff who are helped by alcoholism treatment. 1 photograph.

2.234   "What Industry Is Doing About 10 Million Alcoholic Workers." U.S. News and World Report 80 (January 12, 1976): 66-67.

The cooperative effort of employers, unions, insurance companies and distillers to deal with the problem of employee alcoholism. John Lavino, Jr. (Kemper Insurance Companies) and Dr. Alfred A. Smith (New York Medical College) are two people quoted in this article. 2 photographs.

2.235   Wright, Beric. "Drink, Directors and a Question of Duty." Director 31 (March 1979): 55-56.

A medical adviser talks about the types of drinkers, gives a World Health Organization (WHO) definition of "alcoholic," and comments on the way to deal with this problem in the corporate setting.

2.236   Zepke, Brent E. "Employer Liability for Intoxicated Employees." Supervisory Management 22 (July 1977): 32-39.

A lawyer interprets common and statutory law as they relate to employer liability for intoxicated employees. Author biographical information.

3

Unions, Safety, Employee Dismissal

3.001   "Alcoholism Programs in the Workplace."   Employee Bene-
        fit Plan Review 34 (December 1979):   30 and 107.

        Reports on "Reaching the Alcoholic in the Workplace:
        New Alternatives for the '80s," a one-day seminar. The
        Illinois Chapter of the Association of Labor-Management
        Administrators and Consultants on Alcoholism (ALMACA),
        and the Chicago Federation of Labor and Industrial Union
        Council, AFL-CIO (American Federation of Labor and Con-
        gress of Industrial Organizations) sponsored the semi-
        nar.

3.002   Andrewson, Dale E.   "Arbitral Views of Alcoholism Cases."
        Personnel Journal 58 (May 1979):   318-322.

        This article consists of four main parts: the test of
        just cause, preponderance of evidence, determination
        that an employee is intoxicated, and rehabilitation.   In-
        cludes a chart about contractual clauses and their ef-
        fect on arbitral decision making.   Some of the companies
        listed in the chart: U.S. Steel Corp., DU-CO Ceramics
        Co., Northrop Worldwide Aircraft Services, Inc., Kast
        Metals Corp., Tennessee River Pulp and Paper Co., Pacif-
        ic Northwest Bell Telephone Co., Greenlee Brothers and
        Co., New York Telephone Co., Stokely-Van Camp, Inc., and
        Land O'Lakes Bridgeman Creamery.   Author biographical
        information. 1 chart. 3 references.

3.003   Arner, Oddvar.   "The Role of Alcohol in Fatal Accidents
        among Seamen."   British Journal of Addiction 68 (1973):
        185-189.

        Alcohol is involved in one-third of fatal accidents
        among Norwegian merchant seamen.   This data was presented
        at the Third International Conference on Alcoholism and
        Addictions, Cardiff, September 1970.   Abstract.   Author
        biographical information.   4 references.

3.004   Aronoff, Morton and Henry J. Huestis.   "Smiles or Statis-
        tics--How Are We Doing?:   An Evaluation of the

effectiveness of a Union-Based Occupational Alcoholism
Program in the Broadcast Industry." Labor-Management
Alcoholism Journal 11 (July-August 1981): 26-34.

Morton Aronoff and Henry J. Huestis, employees of the
National Broadcasting Co. (NBC) in New York, administer
a program for alcoholic union members, of the National
Association of Broadcast Employees and Technicians
(NABET). Employees of RCA Records, Reeves-Teletape,
and the National Black Network also belong to the union.
The success of the program is largely attributed to the
many treatment facilities in the New York area. 2 photographs. 2 figures.

3.005   Baer, Walter E.   "Drinking." in Discipline and Discharge under the Labor Agreement, by Walter E. Baer,
79-83. New York, NY: American Management Association,
Inc., 1972.

Circumstances under which an employee may or may not be
dismissed from his job for reasons of alcohol use.

3.006   Bannon, Sharleen. "Alcoholism: A Union-Management Issue." Labour Gazette 75 (July 1975): 419-423.

A feature of this article are photographs of posters
about employees and alcohol abuse at Bethlehem Steel and
General Motors (GM). 3 photographs.

3.007   "Beware: Addicts at Work." Labour Gazette 72 (August
1972): 424-425.

Remarks by Joe Morris, Executive Vice President, Canadian Labour Congress, concerning industrial alcoholism,
and by Dr. Robert G. Wiencek, Medical Director, Detroit
Diesel Allison Division of General Motors (GM).

3.008   Brant, W.G. "Chief." "The King County Labor Council Alcoholism Program." Labor-Management Alcoholism Journal
7 (May-June 1978): 38-40.

The work of the Alcoholism Program of the King County
Labor Council. The alcoholism program, designed and
initiated by James K. Bender, works with labor and management in the Seattle-King County area of Washington
state. Author biographical information. 1 photograph.

3.009   Brechin, Jim. "Union Education in Alcoholism." Canadian Labour 22 (September 1977): 5-7 and 29.

INPUT '77 was the Second Canadian Conference on Occupational Alcoholism and Drug Abuse. INPUT '77 was held
in Toronto during the first week of May 1977. This article is primarily about two speakers at the conference.
Dr. Garry L. Briggs, Director, Member-Counseling Unit,

Alberta Union of Provincial Employees (AUPE), was one of the speakers. The other speaker was Canadian Labour Congress (CLC) Executive Vice-President, Julien Major. Author biographical information.

3.010   Bucky, Steven F. "Effects of Alcohol Abuse on Work Performance." Chapter in The Impact of Alcoholism, by Steven F. Bucky et al, 69-74. Center City, MN: Hazelden, 1978.

Employee tardiness, sick leave, wasted time, accidents, and bad judgements are some of the many effects of alcohol abuse on work performance. Relative to the number of alcoholics in industry, there are extremely few on skid row.

3.011   Burger, Frank P. "Why and How UPIU Is Involved in Backing Alcoholism Programs." Pulp and Paper 51 (March 1977): 103-105.

The work of the United Paperworkers International Union (UPIU) in supporting alcoholism programs for workers. The UPIU first became involved in May 1973. It issued a policy statement in February 1974. Author biographical information. 1 photograph. 1 figure.

3.012   "CLC Programme on Drug and Alcoholism Addiction." Canadian Labour Comment 6 (January 27, 1978): 5.

An interview with Julien Major, Canadian Labour Congress (CLC) Executive Vice-President, indicates the CLC's willingness to combat alcoholism and drug addiction.

3.013   Cole, Gordon H. "Alcoholism: Tragedy on the Job." American Federationist 83 (May 1976): 1-4.

Role of unions in dealing with alcoholism, a thirteen-point union-management policy for establishing an alcoholism treatment program, and a guide for recognizing on-the-job signs of alcoholism. There are four stages of alcoholism--early, middle, late middle, and late--and there are, for each stage, at least nine indicators of alcoholism. Author biographical information. 2 illustrations.

3.014   "Costs of Alcoholism." Labour Gazette 76 (February 1976): 66.

A joint, union-management committee states that employee alcoholism costs the Toronto Transit Commission up to almost $4 million annually. The committee recommended establishment of an employee alcoholism treatment program.

3.015   Coulson, Robert. "The Chronic Alcoholic." in The

Termination Handbook, by Robert Coulson, 94-97. New
York, NY: Free Press, 1981.

Interrelationship between alcoholic employees, employers, and arbitrators.

3.016   Denenberg, Tia Schneider and R.V. Denenberg. "Alco-
        holism and Just Cause for Discharge." Chapter in Al-
        cohol and Drugs: Issues in the Workplace, by Tia
        Schneider Denenberg and R.V. Denenberg, 1-17. Wash-
        ington, DC: Bureau of National Affairs, Inc., 1983.

        A case history of an alcoholic steel company employee
        is used to illustrate the topics covered in this chap-
        ter, including three models of the alcoholic employee
        in arbitration.

3.017   Denenberg, Tia Schneider and R.V. Denenberg. "Equal
        Treatment of the Alcoholic Employee." in Alcohol and
        Drugs: Issues in the Workplace, by Tia Schneider
        Denenberg and R.V. Denenberg, 46-47. Washington, DC:
        Bureau of National Affairs, Inc., 1983.

        Union and company views regarding the discharge of an
        alcoholic meter reader. The union felt this employee
        should have been treated more fairly as had two other
        employees with drinking problems. The latter employees
        were given an opportunity to demonstrate sobriety and
        acceptable behavior. The company stated the meter
        reader--because of his past employment record--did not
        deserve the treatment afforded the other two employees.

3.018   Denenberg, Tia Schneider and R.V. Denenberg. "Reha-
        bilitation Before Discipline?" in Alcohol and Drugs:
        Issues in the Workplace, by Tia Schneider Denenberg and
        R.V. Denenberg, 36-42. Washington, DC: Bureau of Na-
        tional Affairs, Inc., 1983.

        If an employer has an employee assistance program (EAP),
        is that employer obliged to try to rehabilitate an al-
        coholic employee before he disciplines him for deterio-
        rating work performance? One company's policy and an
        arbitrator's findings are examined.

3.019   Denenberg, Tia Schneider and R.V. Denenberg. "Rules on
        Possession and Use of Alcohol." in Alcohol and Drugs:
        Issues in the Workplace, by Tia Schneider Denenberg and
        R.V. Denenberg, 109-110. Washington, DC: Bureau of
        National Affairs, Inc., 1983.

        Discharge of a steel industry employee because he had
        a small amount of alcohol in his locker at work. The
        same day the alcohol was discovered, this employee had
        a serious accident while working. He was found to have
        a high blood alcohol concentration.

3.020   Denenberg, Tia Schneider and R.V. Denenberg. "The Un-
cooperative Employee." in Alcohol and Drugs: Issues
in the Workplace, by Tia Schneider Denenberg and R.V.
Deneberg, 43-45. Washington, DC: Bureau of National
Affairs, Inc., 1983.

A telephone company lineman was discharged from his job
because he refused to fully cooperate with his employer
in the treatment of his alcoholism.

3.021   Eck, William L. "Prevention and Education in the Workplace." Labor-Management Alcoholism Journal 6 (May-
June 1977): 22-23.

Prevention of alcoholism in the workplace can be
achieved through joint union-management programs, which
emphasize early detection and effective motivation to
seek treatment. Author biographical information. 1
photograph.

3.022   Gilstrap, R.W. and E. Paul Hoover. "The Union as a
Catalyst in an Employee Alcoholism Program." Labor-
Management Alcoholism Journal 6 (May-June 1977): 33-38.

The Air Line Pilots Association (ALPA) represents 30,
000 commercial pilots. ALPA, which was formed in 1931,
wants to efficiently deal with alcohol abuse by its
members. ALPA, for this reason, established a Human
Intervention and Motivation Study (HIMS). The National
Institute on Alcohol Abuse and Alcoholism (NIAAA) provided financial assistance. Author biographical information. 6 footnotes.

3.023   Godard, Jacques. "French Approaches to Alcohol Prob-
lems in Employment." Chapter in Alcohol Problems in
Employment, edited by Brian D. Hore and Martin A.
Plant, 173-184. London: Croom Helm Ltd., 1981.

Uses questions and answers directed at employers and
trade unions in France to examine French approaches to
alcohol problems in employment. 1 table.

3.024   Habbe, Stephen. "Controlling the Alcohol Problem: Not
by Management Alone." Conference Board Record 10
(April 1973): 31-33.

Importance of union cooperation with management in
dealing with alcoholic employees. Includes a dialogue
between James F. Horst, Executive Vice President, Trans-
port Workers Union of America, and Marion Sadler, Vice
Chairman, American Airlines. Abstract. Author biographical information. 1 footnote.

3.025   Hibbert, Bill. "One Union's Approach to Alcoholism:
The Seafarers International Union Alcoholism

Rehabilitation Program." Labor-Management Alcoholism
Journal 7 (May-June 1978): 20-21 and 24-27.

The Seafarers Alcoholic Rehabilitation Center in Valley
Lee, Maryland began operation in 1975. A University of
Maryland study had earlier described alcoholism in the
maritime industry. A letter about the union's alcoholism rehabilitation program is included. Author biographical information. 1 photograph.

3.026   Hingson, Ralph W., Ruth I. Lederman and Diana Chapman
Walsh. "Employee Drinking Patterns and Accidental In-
jury: A Study of Four New England States." Journal of
Studies on Alcohol 46 (1985): 298-303.

Employee drinking patterns and accidental injury were
studied in Connecticut, Rhode Island, Vermont, and New
Hampshire. An anonymous telephone survey involved randomly sampled employed adults. Demographic characteristics, drinking behavior, frequency of accidents, and
interrelationships of drinking, drug use, and accidents
are discussed. Author biographical information. Abstract. 1 table. 1 figure. 17 references.

3.027   Hore, Brian D. "Alcohol and Alcoholism: Their Effect
on Work and the Industrial Response." Chapter in Alcohol Problems in Employment, edited by Brian D. Hore and
Martin A. Plant, 10-17. London: Croom Helm Ltd., 1981.

Alcohol affects physiological variables and two problems
in particular--absenteeism and industrial accidents--
arise from worker alcohol abuse. Managing the problem
drinker at work entails overcoming diferent obstacles.
Union and management attitudes can be two of the most
important obstacles to be surmounted.

3.028   Hunt, Richard Earl. "The Impact of Federal Sector Unions
Upon Supervisory Implementation of the Federal Alcoholism
and Equal Employment Opportunity Policies." Dissertation
Abstracts International 42: 877A. Ph.D. dissertation,
Cornell University, 1977. Order No. DA8116576.

This research involved, in part, 651 supervisors, seventy-one federal government installations, twenty-four hypotheses, and interviews with a sample of union leaders.

3.029   "ILO Study on Working Alcoholics." Canadian Labour 18
(March 1973): 32.

The International Labour Organization (ILO) published a
report on alcoholism and drug addiction. Joe Morris,
Canadian Labour Congress (CLC) Executive Vice President,
wrote the report. The report claims that over half the
world's problem drinkers are employed. According to
Morris, an effective rehabilitation program recuires

four conditions.

3.030   Johnson, LeRoy. "Union Responses to Alcoholism." _Journal of Drug Issues_ 11 (1981): 263-277.

Union counseling, union pretreatment referral programs, and local union programs are three examples of unilateral union efforts to fight alcoholism. Limitations--cost and effectiveness--are discussed in relation to these programs. Obtaining program support, referral success, joint union-company programs, and unilateral company programs are also covered. This article ends with issues for unions to face, including federal legislation and making alcoholism programs a bargaining issue. Abstract. Author biographical information. 24 references.

3.031   Kolben, Nancy Sinkin. "Employer and Union-Sponsored Employee Counseling Programs: Trends for the 1980s." _Contemporary Drug Problems_ 11 (1982): 181-201.

Based on a report to the Community Council of Greater New York. New York City is used as a prototype for the rest of the U.S. Data is based on individual interviews. Author biographical information. 16 notes.

3.032   Marmo, Michael. "Arbitrators View Alcoholic Employees: Discipline or Rehabilitation?" _Arbitration Journal_ 37 (March 1982): 17-27.

Progressive discipline and rehabilitation are the two ways that labor and management view treatment of alcoholic employees. Arbitrators have to decide whether to use progressive discipline or rehabilitation, since labor and management often leave this decision to arbitrators. Case studies are included. Author biographical information. Abstract. 2 photographs. 53 footnotes.

3.033   McCann, Colleen. "Discipline or Compassion for an Alcoholic?" _PIMA Magazine_ 67 (April 1985): 13 and 35.

Concerns an arbitrator's decision regarding the termination of an employee of the Coram Paper Mill. The employee was caught intoxicated and driving on company property. 1 photograph.

3.034   McCann, Colleen. "The Price of Beer on Company Premises." _PIMA Magazine_ 66 (August 1984): 25 and 60.

About an employee management dispute at the Tetlor Paper and Pulp Co., concerning the consumption of beer by several staff members at the company. The arbitrator's decision is given. 1 photograph.

3.035   "Morris Outlines Union Role in Addiction Cures." _Canadian Labour_ 17 (March 1972): 21.

Lists five factors which may hinder union cooperation with on-the-job treatment for alcoholics. Joe Morris, Executive Vice President of the Canadian Labour Congress (CLC), spoke about the factors in Vancouver, B.C., at a seminar on alcohol and drugs.

3.036 Nicholson, Richard E. "Of Hooch and Hazards--Alcoholism and Accidents in Industry." Occupational Health Nursing 22 (May 1974): 10-12 and 47.

A paper presented on February 15, 1973 at a seminar in Hartford, Connecticut. The Greater Hartford Chamber of Commerce and the Greater Hartford Council on Alcoholism and Drug Abuse sponsored the seminar. It was entitled "Seminar on Drug Abuse and Alcoholism in Business." Author biographical information. 1 photograph. 19 references.

3.037 Ogden, James B., John Hodges, Robin J. Milstead, James D. Sanders and Joseph H. Mohler. "The Role of Labor in Developing and Utilizing Alcoholism Treatment Facilities." Labor-Management Alcoholism Journal 6 (May-June 1977): 3-21 and 24-32.

Four separate presentations examine the role of labor in developing and utilizing alcoholism treatment facilities. Three labor organizations represented are: the American Federation of Labor and Congress of Industrial Organizations (AFL-CIO), the United Auto Workers (UAW), and the United Steel Workers (USW). Author biographical information. 1 photograph. 3 figures. 1 table. 13 footnotes.

3.038 Older, Harry J., Donald A. Phillips and Arthur J. Purvis. "A New Approach to the Training of Supervisors and Union Personnel." Labor-Management Alcoholism Journal 8 (July-August 1978): 12-21.

A Behavior-Feeling-Behavior (BFB) analysis sensitizes supervisors and union personnel to employee behavior, and affects the feelings and behavior of these supervisors and union personnel, when they deal with alcoholic employees. The BFB analysis may have positive potential in the training of individuals who have to deal with alcoholics, including doctors and social workers, nurses and parole officers. 2 photographs. Author biographical information. 5 footnotes. 2 figures.

3.039 "One Union Viewpoint on PAR." Labor-Management Alcoholism Newsletter 2 (September-October 1972): 16-17.

The American Postal Workers Union, AFL-CIO (American Federation of Labor and Congress of Industrial Organizations) strongly endorses the Program for Alcoholic Recovery (PAR), which provides treatment for alcoholic postal employees.

3.040   Perlis, Leo. "Alcoholism: A Challenge to Labor and
        Management." Labor-Management Alcoholism Journal 7
        (March-April 1978): 17-19 and 23.

        What is known about alcoholism, what is not certain
        about it, and how labor and management can cooperate
        to deal with this problem. 1 photograph.

3.041   Perlis, Leo. "Labor Looks at Alcoholism." Labor-Man-
        agement Alcoholism Newsletter 2 (January-February
        1973): 20-21 and 23.

        The labor viewpoint regarding alcoholism by the Na-
        tional Director, AFL-CIO (American Federation of Labor
        and Congress of Industrial Organizations) Department
        of Community Services. Author biographical informa-
        tion. 1 photograph.

3.042   Perlis, Leo. "Unionism and Alcoholism: The Issues."
        Chapter in Alcoholism and Its Treatment in Industry,
        edited by Carl J. Schramm, 69-74. Baltimore, MD:
        Johns Hopkins University Press, 1977.

        Evolution of labor's position on alcoholism and the
        goals of treatment and rehabilitation.

3.043   "Pipeline Group Works to Limit Alcoholism." Engineer-
        ing News-Record 193 (August 8, 1974): 109.

        Alaska Labor and Management Affairs (ALMEA) is an An-
        chorage, Alaska organization which offers assistance
        to alcoholic pipeline workers. ALMEA is a cooperative
        effort of contractors and unions. Donald Ryder is the
        head of this organization.

3.044   Price, D.L. and R.J. Liddle. "The Effect of Alcohol
        on a Manual Arc Welding Task." Welding Journal 61
        (July 1982): 15-19.

        Twelve male arc welders were the subjects in this study.
        Their ability to work effectively was adversely affect-
        ed when alcohol in their blood reached the 0.09% level.
        The mean age of the welders was 31.7 years. Author
        biographical information. 6 photographs. 1 table. 16
        references.

3.045   Price, Dennis L. and Robert A. Flax. "Alcohol, Task
        Difficulty, and Incentives in Drill Press Operation."
        Human Factors 24 (1982): 573-579.

        Investigates blood alcohol concentration (BAC) levels
        and task difficulty involving drill press operation.
        Eight male subjects--average age twenty-three--took

part in the research. The authors were interested in
speed of production and accuracy in relation to alcohol and performance of drill presses. Author biographical information. Abstract. 4 tables. 2 figures. 6
references.

3.046   Price, Dennis L. and Thomas G. Hicks. "The Effects of
Alcohol on Performance of a Production Assembly Task."
Ergonomics 22 (January 1979): 37-42.

An investigation of blood alcohol and an assembly task,
using male subjects from the Virginia Polytechnic Institute and State University. The researchers were
especially interested in the effects of low levels of
blood alcohol on quality of work errors and number of
units produced. Author biographical information. 2
figures. English, French, and German abstracts. 3
references.

3.047   Provost, Glendel J., Richard C. Stephens, Yvonne F.
Freedman and William R. Smolensky. "Alcohol in the
Workplace: A Review of Recent Arbitration Cases." Employee Relations Law Journal 4 (Winter 1978-1979): 400-
414.

A study of thirty-seven arbitration case reports, representing the time period 1975-1979. Results of the
thirty-seven cases: thirty discharges, six suspensions,
and one reprimand. Staff at the Institute of Labor and
Industrial Relations, University of Houston, did a literature review as the basis for this article. The
thirty-seven notes refer to the arbitration case reports discussed. Abstract. Author biographical information. 1 illustration. 37 notes.

3.048   Sadler, Marion and James F. Horst. "Company/Union Programs for Alcoholics." Harvard Business Review 50
(September-October 1972): 22-24, 26, 28, 30, 34, 152,
154 and 156.

Management and union cooperation is necessary in controlling employee alcoholism. Two cases of an alcoholism control program at American Airlines are examined.
The efforts of American Motors and of the Utah Copper
Division of Kennecott Copper Corp. are also included.
Author biographical information. 1 note. 1 illustration.

3.049   Schachhuber, Dieter. "Local Unions in the Fight against
Alcoholism." Labour Gazette 77 (November 1977): 505-
510.

Why it is in the self-interest of both management and
labor to fight alcoholism. Guidelines are provided for
unions interested in implementing alcoholism programs.

Author biographical information.

3.050   Schlaadt, Richard G. and Peter T. Shannon. "Job-Relat-
        ed Problems." in Drugs of Choice: Current Perspec-
        tives on Drug Use, by Richard G. Schlaadt and Peter T.
        Shannon, Second Edition, 158. Englewood Cliffs, NJ:
        Prentice-Hall, 1986.

        Alcohol consumption and occupational accidents.

3.051   Schramm, Carl J. "Developing Language on Alcoholism
        in Labor-Management Contracts." Monthly Labor Review
        98 (June 1975):   57.

        Makes reference to the four stages pertaining to devel-
        opment of contract language in labor-management con-
        tracts regarding alcoholism. Author biographical in-
        formation.

3.052   Schramm, Carl J. "Development of Comprehensive Lan-
        guage on Alcoholism in Collective Bargaining Agree-
        ments." Journal of Studies on Alcohol 38 (1977):
        1405-1427.

        Includes "Model Contract Language on Alcoholism Pro-
        posed by AFL-CIO." Abstract. Author biographical in-
        formation. 3 tables. 3 references. 1 appendix.

3.053   "Search of Employee." Supervision 40 (April 1978):
        14.

        An arbitrator's ruling concerning the suspension of an
        employee suspected of drinking on the job.

3.054   Seddon, John T., Jr. "The Community Approach to In-
        dustrial Programs." Labor-Management Alcoholism Jour-
        nal 7 (November-December 1977):   35-38.

        The community organization approach to establishing a
        successful industrial alcoholism program entails the
        assistance of top union and corporate leadership. Ad-
        vice on how to approach this leadership is given. Au-
        thor biographical information.

3.055   Shirley, Charles E. "Troubled Programs and Negative
        Attitudes." Labor-Management Alcoholism Journal 9
        (July-August 1979): 2-6.

        Cultural, familial, and experiential factors, in the
        lives of certain key individuals in a corporate or
        union power structure, can account for hidden blocks
        to the implementation of an occupational alcoholism
        program (OAP). Author biographical information.

3.056   Simpson, William S. "Helping Alcoholics Is Good

Business." _Labor-Management Alcoholism Journal_ 4
(September-October 1974):   20-21.

Comparisons are made between company safety programs
and employee alcoholism programs (EAPs), especially
the evolution and gradual acceptance of each. Author biographical information. 1 photograph.

3.057   Smith, Roy W. "Labour and Alcoholism Control." _Cana-
dian Labour_ 19 (September 1974): 24-26.

Role of labor in dealing with alcoholism in Canadian
industry. Emphasizes that alcoholism results in disease, degradation, and death for the compulsive drinker. Also elaborates on five concepts relating to
treating alcoholics: recognition, respect, referral,
reclamation, and readjustment. Author biographical
information.

3.058   Somers, Gerald G. "The Alcoholic Employee." _Employee
Relations Law Journal_ 2 (Summer 1976): 58-65.

Four topics are examined: the growth of occupational
programs for alcoholic employees, collective bargaining approaches to alcoholism, why a union-management
demonstration project is desirable, and evaluation of
alcoholic programs for employees. Author biographical
information. 2 illustrations. 4 notes.

3.059   Spears, John R., Daniel O'Rourke, Floyd L. Stead and
Richard Hartnett. "Evaluating and Monitoring a Union-
Management Occupational Alcoholism Program." _Labor-
Management Alcoholism Journal_ 10 (January-February
1981): 151-160.

Describes the marketing status of the AFL-CIO Appala-
chian Council project in Pennsylvania and Alabama. Author biographical information. 3 figures.

3.060   Trice, Harrison M. and Janice M. Beyer. "A Study of
Union-Management Cooperation in a Long-Standing Alcoholism Program." _Contemporary Drug Problems_ 11 (1982):
295-317.

Union officials were interviewed in nineteen locations
in the U.S. for this study, which was about a corporate, union-management alcoholism program. The study
was funded by a federal grant, a private foundation,
Cornell University, and the State University of New
York at Buffalo. Author biographical information. 2
tables. 21 notes.

3.061   Trice, Harrison M., Richard E. Hunt and Janice M.
Beyer. "Alcoholism Programs in Unionized Work Settings: Problems and Prospects in Union-Management

Cooperation." <u>Journal of Drug Issues</u> 7 (1977): 103-115.

Major areas dealt with: the role played by labor unions in job-based alcoholism policies, labor unions and constructive confrontation, neglect of unions in job-based programs, union initiated and collectively bargained programs, the arbitrator, unions and broad-brush programs, unions and the treatment community, and existing data about labor unions and job-based programs. Author biographical information. Abstract. 44 references.

3.062 Trice, Harrison M. and Paul M. Roman. "On-the-Job Accidents: Impact of Deviant Drinking." in <u>Spirits and Demons at Work: Alcohol and Other Drugs on the Job</u>, by Harrison M. Trice and Paul M. Roman, Second Edition, 141-144. Ithaca, NY: New York State School of Industrial and Labor Relations Cornell University, 1978.

The authors claim that on-the-job accidents of deviant drinkers are fewer in number than that commonly be-lieved. The authors talk about this in relation to a number of factors, including alcoholics, nonalcoholics, neurotics, psychotics, and normal people.

3.063 Tucker, Jerry R. "A Worker-Oriented Alcoholism and 'Troubled Employee' Program: A Union Approach." <u>In-dustrial Gerontology: New Series</u> 1 (Fall 1974): 20-24.

A union alcoholism program in Missouri. The program--it began in April 1973--is available to over half a million trade union members in that state. The program has offices in St. Louis and Kansas City. Author bio-graphical information. 1 reference.

3.064 "A Union-Based Program for Smaller Employers." <u>Labor-Management Alcoholism Journal</u> 8 (September-October 1978): 45-57.

Dr. Eugene Silbermann was instrumental in the establish-ment of an employee alcoholism program (EAP) for Local 338 of the Retail, Wholesale, and Chain Store Food Em-ployees Union. Local 338 represents 600 individual employers and 15,000 members in New York and parts of Long Island. A few of the 600 individual employers include: Associated Retail Stores, Inc., Duro Mar-kets, Inc., Food City Markets, Inc., Great-Way Foods, Inc., Royal Farms Supermarkets, Shopwell, Inc., and Sloan's Supermarkets, Inc. 7 photographs. 2 foot-notes.

3.065 "Union Role in Rehabilitation of Alcoholics."

Canadian Labour 19 (September 1974): 26.

Remarks by Canadian Labour Congress (CLC) President,
Joe Morris, about on-the-job assistance for alcohol-
ics. The remarks were made in Vancouver, B.C. at a
seminar on alcohol and drugs. The B.C. Workmen's
Compensation Board and the Alcoholism and Narcotics
Addiction Foundation sponsored the seminar.

3.066 Weinstein, Ted. "Lloyd Fell's Lifeline from Alcoholic
       Oblivion." Labour Gazette 75 (April 1975): 239-242.

       Lloyd Fell is a former alcoholic who was treated for
       his condition at the Donwood Institute in Toronto.
       Fell, employed in Toronto by the United Steel Workers
       of America, established Operation Lifeline. It is a
       non-profit organization which assists people who are
       alcoholics or drug addicts. The Continental Can Co.
       of Canada Ltd. is a company whose cooperation with
       Lifeline dates back to Lifeline's inception. Author
       biographical information. 2 photographs.

3.067 Weiss, Richard M. "The Role of Unions." Chapter in
       Dealing with Alcoholism in the Workplace, by Richard
       M. Weiss, 41-51. New York, NY: Conference Board,
       Inc., 1980.

       Joint union-management programs, union involvement and
       program structures, and union involvement and program
       processes and outcomes are the three major topics cov-
       ered. Examples of a grievance procedure and union-man-
       agement correspondence on a problem employee are given.
       4 exhibits. 4 tables.

3.068 Whincup, Michael. "Case Studies 20 and 21." in Law
       and Practice of Dismissal in the Health Service: The
       General Principles of Law and Twenty-Five N.H.S. Case
       Studies, by Michael Whincup, 103-106. Kent: Ravenwood,
       1982.

       Dismissal for drunkenness of a hospital porter, senior
       nursing officer, and a volunteer fireman in Britain.

3.069 White, A.C. "The Relationship between Alcohol and In-
       dustrial Accidents." British Journal on Alcohol and
       Alcoholism 12 (Winter 1977): 165-166.

       Data for this research was obtained from the Birming-
       ham (England) Accident Hospital Burns Unit. The data
       pertains to the time period May 1975 to May 1976.
       Fifty-six industrial accident victims, divided into
       two groups of twenty-eight, participated in the re-
       search. One group consisted of patients who were un-
       likely to have contributed to their accidents; the
       second group was made up of patients who might have

contributed to their accidents. Alcohol impairment
was related to industrial accidents. Author biographical information. 1 table. 4 references.

3.070   Wolkenberg, Robert C., Calman Gold and Erwin R.
        Tichauer. "Delayed Effects of Acute Alcoholic Intox-
        ication on Performance with Reference to Work Safe-
        ty." Journal of Safety Research 7 (September 1975):
        104-118.

        A simulated industrial work situation was the setting
        for this study. Nine male subjects who engaged in an
        evening of social drinking were the population sample.
        Lengthened reaction time and decreased motor sensory
        skill were two of the aftereffects of alcohol on the
        subjects. Abstract. Author biographical information.
        9 figures. 2 tables. 34 references.

4

Government

4.001   Ajas, Hiroshi. "USAF Alcohol Abuse Control: Does It
        Meet the Needs of the Military Family?" Government
        Reports Announcements and Index 86 (August 1, 1986):
        38. NTIS AD-A166 673/4/GAR.

        The U.S. Air Force has resources to provide assis-
        tance to military alcoholics and their families. How-
        ever, greater efforts should be made to better inform
        these alcoholics, spouses, and families about the
        available treatment and counseling services. 6 ta-
        bles. 74 references.

4.002   "Alcoholism Programs." Labour Gazette 76 (January
        1976): 10.

        Speaking at a conference on occupational health and
        drug abuse, Marc Lalonde, Canada's Health Minister,
        said more Canadian companies should have employee al-
        coholism treatment programs. S.C.M. Ambler, Chairman
        of the Ontario Division, Canadian Manufacturers' Asso-
        ciation, claims most companies cannot afford these
        programs.

4.003   "Amtrak Program Described." Labor-Management Alcohol-
        ism Journal 10 (May-June 1981): 246-250.

        Remarks of Robert T. Eckenrode, Group Vice President
        for Finance and Administration, National Railroad Pas-
        senger Corp. He spoke about the Amtrak employee as-
        sistance program (EAP), when he addressed the Labor-
        Management Luncheon of the National Council on Alco-
        holism (NCA) Annual Forum. 1 photograph.

4.004   Armor, David J., Bruce R. Orvis, Polly Carpenter-Huff-
        man and J. Michael Polich. "The Control of Alcohol
        Problems in the U.S. Air Force." Government Reports
        Announcements and Index 82 (August 13, 1982): 3382.
        NTIS AD-A113 797/5.

        Concentrates on five areas: the prevalence of alcohol

problems, effectiveness of alcohol education, identification and treatment, cost effectiveness of the
control program, and policy options for the air
force. Abstract. 5 figures. 6 tables. 17 references.

4.005   Babayan, E.A. and M.H. Gonopolsky. Textbook on Al-
        coholism and Drug Abuse in the Soviet Union. New
        York, NY: International Universities Press, Inc.,
        1985.

        English translation of a book published in Russian.
        Thirty-nine chapters cover the Soviet substance abuse
        service, which includes a campaign against heavy
        drinking and alcoholism. Clinical, social, and legal
        aspects are examined. Methods of therapy are dis-
        cussed. 4 figures. 4 tables. 5 diagrams.

4.006   Babor, Thomas F., Michel Treffardier, Jacques Weill,
        Luc Fegueur and J.P. Ferrant. "The Early Detection
        and Secondary Prevention of Alcoholism in France."
        Journal of Studies on Alcohol 44 (1983): 600-616.

        Covered are: background, treatment assumptions and
        procedures, ethical issues in recruitment and screen-
        ing, reliability and validity of the grid method, and
        program effectiveness. Employment and alcoholism are
        included, particularly railroad workers. Author bio-
        graphical information. Abstract. 1 figure. 1 ta-
        ble. 4 footnotes. 22 references.

4.007   Bailar, Benjamin Franklin. "PAR Philosophy Reflected
        in Program." Labor-Management Alcoholism Journal 7
        (March-April): 1978: 20-22.

        The U.S. Postal Service established in 1969, in San
        Francisco, the first Program for Alcoholic Recovery
        (PAR) unit for postal employees. Nine years later,
        in 1978, there were 122 PAR offices coast-to-coast.
        The PAR success rate is 75%. Author biographical in-
        formation. 1 photograph.

4.008   Balunov, O.A. and Bernard Segal. "Development and
        Organization of Services for Alcoholics in Leningrad,
        U.S.S.R." International Journal of the Addictions
        21 (1986): 97-103.

        One Russian and one American are the coauthors of
        this article. It mentions alcoholism and the work-
        place. Author biographical information. Abstract.
        10 notes.

4.009   Borthwick, R.B. "Summary of Cost-Benefit Study Re-
        sults for Navy Alcoholism Rehabilitation Programs."
        Government Reports Announcements and Index 77

(October 28, 1977):   56.   NTIS AD-A042 795/5GA.

The economic cost of alcohol abuse in the U.S. is $32
billion annually. The figure for the Department of
the Navy ranges between $360 million and $680 each
year. It is much more economic to the navy to rehabilitate alcoholic personnel than to replace them
with new personnel. Eighty-three percent of navy alcoholics age twenty-six and over are treated successfully. Abstract. 8 figures. 5 tables.

4.010   Bucky, Steven F., Darrel Edwards and Newell H. Berry.
"A Note on Hospitalization and Discharge Rates of Men
Treated at the Navy's Alcohol Center." Government
Reports Announcements and Index 80 (February 29, 1980):
732. NTIS AD-A077 157/6

Two pilot studies revealed that treatment was very
successful for alcoholics in the navy. An indicator
of successful treatment in the second study was a very
dramatic decrease in the number of sick days after
treatment. Author biographical information. Abstract.
1 reference. 2 footnotes.

4.011   Burgess, C. Duane and Anne D. Robertson. "The Missis-
sippi Plan for Community Alcoholism Treatment." in
Aspects of Alcohol and Drug Dependence, edited by J.S.
Madden, Robin Walker and W.H. Kenyon, 332-336. Kent:
Pitman Medical Ltd., 1980.

Distilled spirits and wine were not legally sold, pur-
chased, or consumed in Mississippi prior to 1966. In
1980 approximately 50% of Mississippi was still "dry."
County and municipality option on the sale of distilled spirits and wine helps regulate in which parts of
the state these beverages are sold. The Mississippi
Division of Alcohol and Drug Abuse, within the Department of Mental Health, is responsible for treatment
services. Regional halfway houses, regional detoxification services, and vocational rehabilitation programs are some of the treatment services available.
This paper is based on the Proceedings of the Fourth
International Conference on Alcoholism and Drug Dependence, Liverpool, England.

4.012   Butler, Elizabeth M. Alcoholism Programs in Industry:
An Alberta Survey. Edmonton: Alberta Workers' Health,
Safety and Compensation, 1982.

One thousand industries in Alberta were surveyed via
questionnaire in order to examine industrial alcohol
abuse and its treatment. The questionnaire response
rate was 57.6%. Thirty-three of the 576 respondents
were subsequently interviewed. This study includes
seven recommendations. 27 tables. 5 figures. 82

references.   5 appendices.

4.013   Butynski, W.   "Status of State Legislation and Re-
search on Health Insurance Coverage for Alcoholism
Treatment." <u>Government Reports Announcements and
Index</u> 83 (January 21, 1983):   234. NTIS PB83-111526.

Contains some information about employers, unions
alcoholism, and self-insurance.

4.014   Cahalan, Don and Ira Cisin.   "Attitudes and Behavior
of Naval Personnel Concerning Alcohol and Problem
Drinking." <u>Government Reports Announcements and In-
dex</u> 77 (April 1, 1977):   34. NTIS AD-A034821.

This study was conducted for the U.S. Navy Department
Bureau of Naval Personnel by the Bureau of Social Science Research, Inc., Washington, D.C. Over 1600 officers and enlisted men were surveyed. The study
gives the methods utilized, defines and measures
drinking problems and drinking behavior, compares the
findings of mail and field-administered questionnaires,
compares results for officers and enlisted men, compares results for four types of sample sites, and gives
recommendations for further research. 18 footnotes.
30 tables. 3 appendices.

4.015   Cahalan, Don and Ira H. Cisin.   "Final Report on a
Service-Wide Survey of Attitudes and Behavior of Naval
Personnel Concerning Alcohol and Problem Drinking."
<u>Government Reports Announcements and Index</u> 75 (October
3, 1975):   30. NTIS AD-A013 236/5GA.

A mail survey was used to sample 9508 male and female
personnel on active duty in the U.S. Navy. Five main
areas studied included: drinking practices and problems among naval personnel, job-connected drinking
problems, the navy drinking climate, attitudes and experiences concerning prevention and treatment, and navy drinking compared to civilian drinking. Author
biographical information. Abstract. 40 tables. 4
appendices.

4.016   Cahalan, Don, Ira H. Cisin, Geoffrey L. Gardner and
Gorman C. Smith.   "Drinking Practices and Problems in
the U.S. Army, 1972." <u>Government Reports Announcements and Index</u> 73 (September 25, 1973):   19. NTIS
AD-763 851.

Compares the drinking practices and problems of male
U.S. Army personnel to the drinking practices and
problems of civilians. A random sample of nearly 10,
000 army personnel were surveyed via questionnaire.
The report discusses: how the study was done, army-

civilian comparisons, comparisons among pay grade, direct costs of alcohol abuse, the army drinking climate, drinking behavior within geographic areas, and a multivariate analysis of the army problem drinking. Author biographical information. Abstract. 6 appendices. 35 tables. 3 figures.

4.017 California Office of Alcoholism. "California Alcoholism Program: 1977 Report to the Legislature." Government Reports Announcements and Index 78 (February 3, 1978): 36. NTIS PB-273 999/3GA.

Includes information about alcoholism and employment.

4.018 Canada. Treasury Board. Personnel Policy Branch. Occupational Health and Safety Group. Alcohol Dependence and Work Performance. Ottawa: Minister of Supply and Services, 1978.

A pamphlet which describes the Employee Assistance Program (EAP) available to members of the Canadian Public Service, who have drinking problems. The program was announced by the Treasury Board in October 1977. 1 appendix.

4.019 Cocke, Eugene R. "The Control of Alcoholism in Combat Arms Units." Government Reports Announcements and Index 73 (July 25, 1973): 51. NTIS AD-760 918.

Differentiates between alcohol abuse, alcoholic, alcoholism, and problem drinker. Looks at the impact of alcohol, including alcohol abuse and the military; discusses specific problems, for example, alcohol problem identification; and elaborates on a tactical unit approach. Lists seven conclusions and makes seven recommendations. Author biographical information. Abstract. 55 footnotes. 2 figures. 60 references. 1 appendix.

4.020 Connecticut State Alcohol Council. "Connecticut Action Plan for Alcoholism Prevention and Treatment 1976." Government Reports Announcements and Index 77 (February 18, 1977): 46-47. NTIS HRP-0012179/8GA.

Includes information about occupational alcoholism. 6 footnotes. 13 appendices. 18 tables. 3 maps.

4.021 Cosper, Ronald Lee. "Drinking among Naval Aviators: Patterns of Alcohol Use in an Occupational Specialty." Dissertation Abstracts International 37: 3921A. Ph.D. dissertation, Rutgers University (New Brunswick), 1976. Order No. DA7626994.

Although alcohol use has often been viewed as a deviance, this dissertation questions that view. In the

military, a subculture of heavy drinking provides re-
wards for difficult conditions. A questionnaire was
used to obtain data on the drinking practices of eighty-
four naval aviators. Their heavy drinking was not seen
as pathological. Furthermore, it cannot be explained
in terms of numerous variables, including age, social
class, and religion.

4.022   Durning, Kathleen P. and Erik Jansen. "Problem Drinking and Attitudes toward Alcohol among Navy Recruits."
Government Reports Announcements and Index 76 (February 20, 1976): 25. NTIS AD-A018 754/2GA.

The sample for this research were over 2000 male navy
recruits, who entered basic training at the Recruit
Training Command in San Diego, California. The recruits were administered an alcohol experiences questionnaire. It was very common for navy recruits to
have had problems with alcohol prior to enlisting in
the navy. Author biographical information. Abstract.
4 tables. 11 references. 2 appendices.

4.023   Edwards, Darrel, Virginia Iorio, Newell H. Berry and
E.K. Eric Gunderson. "Prediction of Success for Al-
coholics in the Navy: A First Look." Journal of
Clinical Psychology 29 (January 1973): 86-89.

Data pertaining to nearly 5000 navy male patients, at
thirty-one naval hospitals, was used in this investigation. The results of the investigation concerned:
a comparison of alcoholic patients with all other psychiatric patients, length of hospitalization and dis-
position, correlates of the return to duty (RTD) dis-
position for alcoholic patients, and correlates of successful posthospital adjustment. Author biographical
information. 2 tables. 1 reference.

4.024   Eringer, Robert. "Down the Hatch." Harper's 266
(April 1983): 16-17

Reports on drinking problems among enlisted men and
commissioned officers in the U.S. Navy. U.S. Service-
men worldwide can purchase alcoholic beverages at extremely low prices at any U.S. military base. Treatment facilities are located in Britain and throughout
parts of continental Europe. Author biographical information. 1 cartoon illustration.

4.025   Favazza, Armando R. and Jeannine Pires. "The Michigan
Alcoholism Screening Test: Application in a General
Military Hospital." Quarterly Journal of Studies on
Alcohol 35 (1974): 925-929.

Two hundred and fifty-eight enlisted Navy men, divided
into four groups, were the research sample for this

investigation. All the men were under age forty and
were administered the Michigan Alcoholism Screening
Test (MAST). MAST scores are discussed for each of the
four groups of subjects. Author biographical information. Abstract. 2 tables. 4 references.

4.026 "The Fight That Can Be Won." Labor-Management Alcoholism Newsletter 2 (January-February 1973): 29-30.

Excerpts from "Alcoholism in America--The Fight That
Can Be Won," a speech by Senator Harold E. Hughes. The
Iowa Democrat addressed the National Press Club in Wash-
ington, D.C. in January 1973.

4.027 Fiman, Byron G., Daryl R. Conner and A. Carl Segal. "A
Comprehensive Alcoholism Program in the Army." American Journal of Psychiatry 130 (May 1973): 532-535.

Describes a comprehensive alcoholism program in the U.S.
Army. The origin of the program, developed at Fort
Benning, Georgia, dates back to 1967. A variety of
therapies, staff education and development, and civilian
and military attitudinal changes toward alcoholism were
three reasons given for the program's success. Abstract.
Author biographical information. 16 references.

4.028 Fitzgibbon, Constantine. "Appendix I: Alcoholism and
the Industrial Worker." in Drink, by Constantine Fitzgibbon, 163-168. London: Granada Publishing Ltd., 1980.

This appendix is by the Irish National Council on Alcoholism. The appendix was originally in a report to the
Government of the Republic of Ireland. The report resulted from an international conference on alcoholism
held in Ireland in 1971.

4.029 Ford, Michael. "NCA Fights Efforts to Diminish Rehabilitation Act Safeguards." Labor-Management Alcoholism
Journal 8 (September-October 1978): 57-61.

Letters were sent by the National Council on Alcoholism
(NCA) to two U.S. senators. The letters were about legislation which would exclude alcoholics requiring rehabilitation from anti-discrimination provisions of the
1973 Rehabilitation Act. The senators to whom the letters were addressed: Harrison Williams, Jr. (Democrat-
New Jersey) and Jennings Randolph (Democrat-West Virginia). Williams is Chairman, Human Resources Committee.
Randolph is Chairman, Human Resources Subcommittee on
the Handicapped. Author biographical information.

4.030 Glass, George S. "The Alcohol Rehabilitation Unit, National Naval Medical Center, Bethesda." Military Medicine 139 (June 1974): 486-488.

The alcoholism treatment program at the National Naval
Medical Center in Bethesda, Maryland consists of: individual counseling, an educational program, group meetings, Alcoholics Anonymous (AA), antabuse, ancillary
treatment, and follow-up for discharged patients.   The
Alcohol Rehabilitation Unit is comprised of three services: inpatient service, hospital-wide consultation
service, and outpatient service.   Author biographical
information.   8 references.

4.031   Godwin, Donald F.   "New Directions in Occupational Pro-
        grams for NIAAA."   Labor-Management Alcoholism Journal
        7 (July-August 1977):   39-43.

        National Institute on Alcohol Abuse and Alcoholism
        (NIAAA) funding priorities are discussed.   Included is
        a description of four occupational alcoholism treatment
        models: the in-house program, the OPC (occupational
        program consultant) effort, the consortium, and the
        treatment center outreach program.   Author biographical
        information.   1 photograph.

4.032   Groeneveld, Judith, Martin Shain, Donald Brayshaw and
        Isabel Heideman.   The Alcoholism Treatment Program at
        Canadian National Railways: A Case Study.   Toronto:
        Addiction Research Foundation, 1984.

        Canadian National Railways (CNR) developed and implemented
        an alcoholism treatment program in 1971.   This publica-
        tion is an evaluation of that program.   Approximately 900
        Canadian National (CN) employees took part in the evalu-
        ation.   73 tables.   1 figure.   8 references.   1 appendix.

4.033   Gunderson, E.K. Eric and Marc A. Schuckit.   "Hospital-
        ization Rates for Alcoholism in the Navy and Marine
        Corps."   Government Reports Announcements and Index 77
        (June 10, 1977):   63.   NTIS AD-A037 474/4GA.

        The first of a series of reports on alcoholism in the
        U.S. Navy.   The authors feel that the findings discussed
        in the series may also be of value to research in indus-
        try.   2 figures.   1 table.   Abstract.

4.034   Gwinner, P.D.V.   "The Treatment of Alcoholics in a Mili-
        tary Context."   Journal of Alcoholism 11 (Spring 1976):
        24-31.

        This article was originally presented in 1975 at an al-
        cohol abuse lecture.   Author biographical information.
        5 tables.   1 diagram.   4 references.

4.035   Halloran, Barney.   "Juice."   Soldiers 27 (October 1972):
        4-12.

        Alcohol abuse and the U.S. soldier.   5 photographs.   5

exhibits.

4.036   Hauge, Christian Francis. "Description and Evaluation
of Centralized Alcohol Rehabilitation Programs, United
States Air Force." Dissertation Abstracts International
40: 3535A-3536A. D.S.W. dissertation, University of
Utah, 1979. Order No. DA7927076.

Ten alcohol treatment centers comprise Centralized Alcohol Treatment in the U.S. Air Force. A total of 119
patients and staff were the subjects of study. Research
instruments used included the Sixteen Personality Factor Questionnaire, State-Trait Anxiety Inventory, and
the Community-Oriented Programs Environment Scale.

4.037   Heckman, Norma A., Douglas Kolb and John G. Looney.
"Prevalence of Alcoholism among Navy Hospital Inpa-
tients." Government Reports Announcements and Index 81
(November 6, 1981): 4855-4856. NTIS AD-A101 511/4.

The Brief MAST Test was used to test male patients in a
naval hospital. The patients were divided into three
groups: alcoholic, questionable alcoholic, and nonalcoholic. MAST scores revealed about half of the patients
to be either alcoholic or questionable alcoholic. Author biographical information. 11 references. Abstract.

4.038   Hoiberg, A. and C. Blood. "Health Risks of Diving among
U.S. Navy Officers." Government Reports Announcements
and Index 86 (January 31, 1986): 38. NTIS AD-A160 588/
0/GAR.

Alcoholism was one variable studied in research which
compared diving to nondiving U.S. navy officers. Author
biographical information. 14 references. 2 tables. Abstract.

4.039   Hoiberg, Anne, Steven P. Berard and John Ernst. "Racial
Differences in Hospitalization Rates among Navy Enlisted
Men." Public Health Reports 96 (March-April 1981): 121-
127.

Medical data for hospitalized, U.S. Navy enlisted men,
throughout the world, was obtained from the Navy Medical
Data Services Center in Bethesda, Maryland. This data
was studied at the Naval Health Research Center in San
Diego, California. The enlisted men were categorized as:
White, Black, Malaysian, American Indian or Asian-Ameri-
can. The majority of hospitalizations for alcoholism
was among American Indians. Author biographical information. 3 tables. 1 figure. 2 footnotes. 17 references.

4.040   Holcomb, James F. "Alcohol and the Armed Forces." Alcohol Health and Research World 6 (Winter 1981-1982): 2-
17.

Areas covered include: the prevalence of alcohol use, quantity of alcohol consumed during a typical drinking day, the adverse physiological effects of alcohol, alcohol dependence, consequences of alcohol use, work impairment because of alcohol use, comparison of alcohol use between military personnel and civilians, reasons for not using alcohol, and reasons for using it. Author biographical information. 1 illustration. 15 tables. 4 references. 5 footnotes.

4.041   Holder, H.D., J.O. Blose and M.J. Gasiorowski. "Alcoholism Treatment Impact on Total Health Care Utilization and Costs: A Four-Year Longitudinal Analysis of the Federal Employees Health Benefit Program with Aetna Life Insurance Company." Government Reports Announcements and Index 86 (June 20, 1986): 52. NTIS PB86-181757/GAR.

This study revealed that, in a comparison of alcoholic and nonalcoholic families, the alcoholic families used health care services and incurred costs at twice the rate of nonalcoholic families. 124 footnotes. 72 tables. 14 figures. 1 exhibit. 12 references. 7 appendices.

4.042   Illinois State Department of Mental Health and Developmental Disabilities. "State of Illinois Plan for the Treatment and Prevention of Alcohol Abuse and Alcoholism for Illinois Fiscal Years, 1978-1980." Government Reports Announcements and Index 78 (September 15, 1978): 40. NTIS PB-282 405/OGA.

Parts of this report are about occupational programs for alcoholic employees.

4.043   Killeen, John E. "Military Intervention Programs." Chapter in Prevention of Alcohol Abuse, edited by Peter M. Miller and Ted D. Nirenberg, 469-502. New York, NY: Plenum Press, 1984.

There are six main topics covered regarding Department of Defense, alcohol abuse intervention programs: the target of prevention, the characteristics of alcohol abuse in the military, rationale for the existent problem, difficulties in attacking alcohol abuse, review of current programs, and evaluation of these programs. Author biographical information. 13 tables. 34 references.

4.044   Knowlton, Paul B. and Dale L. Zeller. "The Changing Attitudes on Alcoholism in the Air Force: A Study on Current Attitudes of Military Supervisors." Government Reports Announcements and Index 77 (March 4, 1977): 42. NTIS AD-A032 535/7GA.

This publication is a master's thesis presented by the two authors to the Faculty of the School of Systems and Logistics, Air Force Institute of Technology Air University. Author biographical information. Abstract. 10 tables. 1 appendix. 43 references.

4.045   Kolb, D. and E.K.E. Gunderson. "Research on Alcohol Abuse and Rehabilitation in the U.S. Navy." <u>Government Reports Announcements and Index</u> 84 (February 17, 1984): 65. NTIS AD-A134 897/8.

Data from the Naval Health Research Center in San Diego, California was used in this report. Four alcoholism treatment programs are compared: centers (nonmedical residential), services (medical residential), drydocks or Counseling and Assistance Centers (short-term residential or outpatient), and the Navy Alcohol Safety Action Program (after-hours educational program). Author biographical information. Abstract. 7 references. 4 tables.

4.046   Kolb, Douglas, Gregory D. Baker and E.K. Eric Gunderson. "Effects of Alcohol Rehabilitation Treatment on Health and Performance of Navy Enlisted Men." <u>Government Reports Announcements and Index</u> 83 (February 4, 1983): 415. NTIS AD-A120 038/5.

A group of navy enlisted men, who abused alcohol, were compared to two control groups. An alcohol rehabilitation program the navy enlisted men took part in had a beneficial effect on their post-treatment health and performance. 2 tables. 3 figures. Abstract.

4.047   Kolb, Douglas, Patricia Cohen and E.K. Eric Gunderson. "Comparisons of the Navy Alcohol Safety Action Program with Other Alcohol Rehabilitation Programs." <u>Government Reports Announcements and Index</u> 80 (September 12, 1980): 3916. NTIS AD-A085 119/6.

The Navy Alcohol Safety Action Program (NASAP), when compared with other alcohol rehabilitation programs, rated very highly. 5 tables. 1 reference. 2 appendices. Abstract.

4.048   Kolb, Douglas and E.K. Eric Gunderson. "Alcohol-Related Morbidity among Older Career Navy Men." <u>Government Reports Announcements and Index</u> 82 (May 21, 1982): 2071. NTIS AD-A110 414/0.

Older career navy men, who are alcohol abusers, are compared to a control group. Comparisons are made in a number of ways, including: mean numbers of hospital admissions in thirteen time periods and hospitalization rates during the second half of a navy career. Data maintained at the Naval Health Research Center in San

Diego, California was used. Author biographical information. 4 tables. 17 references. Abstract.

4.049 Kolb, Douglas and E.K. Eric Gunderson. "A Longitudinal Study of Health Risks Associated with Alcohol Abuse in Young Navy Men." Government Reports Announcements and Index 81 (November 6, 1981): 4856. NTIS AD-A101 787/0.

A navy alcohol abuse group, when compared to a control group, was more frequently hospitalized for conditions other than alcoholism than was the control group. Poisonings, infective and parasitic diseases, and diseases of the digestive system were reasons for hospitalization. Author biographical information. 4 tables. 19 references. Abstract.

4.050 Kolb, Douglas and E.K. Eric Gunderson. "Medical Histories of Alcohol Abusers and Controls During the First Twelve Years of Naval Service." Government Reports Announcements and Index 81 (November 6, 1981): 4856. NTIS AD-A101 790/4.

This study revealed that a higher number of alcohol abusers than controls were hospitalized. Hospital admission history data was used in the research. Three common reasons for hospitalization included accidents, violence, and respiratory system disease. Abstract. Author biographical information. 5 tables. 26 references.

4.051 Kolb, Douglas, E.K. Eric Gunderson and Steven Bucky. "Effectiveness of Treatment for Navy Enlisted Men in Alcohol Rehabilitation Centers and Units." Government Reports Announcements and Index 75 (October 3, 1975): 29. NTIS AD-A013 061/7GA.

The authors, affiliated with the Navy Alcoholic Rehabilitation Center Naval Station in San Diego, California, prepared this report for the Department of the Navy Bureau of Medicine and Surgery. The subjects of research were navy enlisted men who were admitted to four Alcohol Rehabilitation Centers and fourteen Alcohol Rehabilitation Units. Treatment effectiveness of individual centers and units is compared. Author biographical information. Abstract. 3 tables. 4 references.

4.052 Kolb, Douglas and E.K.E. Gunderson. "Prognostic Indicators for Navy Alcoholics in Rehabilitation Centers and Units." Government Reports Announcements and Index 75 (June 27, 1975): 35. NTIS AD-A009 089/4GA.

The post-treatment success of two age groups of navy alcoholics were compared. Age twenty-five and younger were designated as the young category. Age twenty-six

and older were designated as the old category. There
were over 2700 subjects in the study. Author biographical information. Abstract. 4 references. 4 footnotes. 3 tables.

4.053   Krebs, James M. "New Directions for Army Alcohol and
Drug Abuse Control." Government Reports Announcements
and Index 76 (April 30, 1976): 75. NTIS AD-A021 646/
5GA.

Discusses the evolution of the U.S. Army alcohol and
drug abuse program. Prevention, identification, treatment, and rehabilitation are also discussed. Author
biographical information. Abstract. 70 footnotes. 37
references.

4.054   Kruzich, David J., Tomi MacDonough, Michael Hawkins
and Harry D. Silsby. "Alcoholism Treatment Outcomes
among Career Soldiers." International Journal of the
Addictions 21 (1986): 139-145.

The research setting for this investigation was the William Beaumont Army Medical Center (WBAMC) Alcoholism
Residential Treatment Facility (ARTF) in El Paso, Texas. The facility opened in 1980 and the subjects of
study included patients admitted from November 1980 to
December 1981. Among the variables studied were: age,
years of education, Michigan Alcoholism Screening Test
(MAST) score, prior Alcoholics Anonymous (AA) contact,
and marital status. The overall success rate of the
treatment program was 77%. Author biographical information. Abstract. 2 tables. 8 references.

4.055   Larkins, Richard D. "Alcohol Misuse among USAF Civilian Employees." Government Reports Announcements and
Index 80 (February 29, 1980): 723. NTIS AD-A076 455/5.

This publication is a master's thesis presented to the
Faculty of the School of Engineering, Air Force Institute of Technology Air University. Of the 110 hypotheses tested for this thesis, sixty-five hypotheses were
supported. Author biographical information. Abstract.
9 figures. 35 tables. 30 references.

4.056   Lewis, Jay. "The Federal Alcoholism Effort." American
Pharmacy NS 22 (April 1982): 10-11.

A look at federal legislation in 1981 regarding alcoholism in the U.S., and what will likely be important alcoholism legislation in 1982. The names of federal agencies, legislators, and statistics are given. Author
biographical information.

4.057   Lewis, Jay. "The Federal Role in Alcoholism Research,
Treatment and Prevention." Chapter in Alcohol, Science

and Society Revisited, edited by Edith Lisansky Gomberg, Helene Raskin White and John A. Carpenter, 385-401. Ann Arbor, MI: University of Michigan Press, 1982.

The Hughes Act of 1970 created the National Institute on Alcohol Abuse and Alcoholism (NIAAA). This chapter is about the political and economic influences which have affected the NIAAA since 1970. An epilogue views the NIAAA within the context of the Reagan election victory of November 1980. 3 footnotes. 40 references.

4.058   Los Angeles Mayor Announces Program for City Employees." Labor-Management Alcoholism Journal 4 (January-February 1975): 42-43.

Establishment of an alcoholism program for employees of the City of Los Angeles. The text of a memorandum by Los Angeles Mayor Tom Bradley, describing the program, is included in this article.

4.059   Maine Office of Alcoholism and Drug Abuse Prevention. "Five-Year Forward Plan for Comprehensive Alcoholism Services for Maine." Government Reports Announcements and Index 78 (March 3, 1978): 42. NTIS PB-274 549/5GA.

Appendix A is about a proposal for a state occupational program for alcoholic employees.

4.060   Manley, T. Roger, Charles W. McNichols and Michael J. Stahl. "Alcoholism and Alcohol Related Problems among USAF Civilian Employees." Government Reports Announcements and Index 80 (February 29, 1980): 723. NTIS AD-A076 599/0.

Nearly 10,000 U.S. Air Force civilian employees were randomly selected and completed a questionnaire regarding alcohol related problems. Prevalence rates, job impact, and psychological dependence are the three areas focused on most extensively in this study. Author biographical information. Abstract. 47 tables. 34 references.

4.061   Mannello, T.A. and F.J. Seaman. "Prevalence, Costs, and Handling of Drinking Problems on Seven Railroads." Government Reports Announcements and Index 81 (April 10, 1981): 1499. NTIS PB81-132516.

The authors, who are with the University Research Corp. in Washington, D.C., prepared this report for the U.S. Federal Railroad Administration (FRA). Project REAP (Railroad Employee Assistance Project) is the subject of the report. REAP dealt with alcohol abuse in the railroad industry. Management and labor personnel cooperated in the research. Over 6000, randomly selected railroad employees completed mailed questionnaires. Abstract.

List of abbreviations. Glossary. 2 appendices. 9 figures. 81 tables. 230 references.

4.062   Matsunaga, Spark. "The Federal Role in Research, Treat-
        ment, and Prevention of Alcoholism." American Psychol-
        ogist 38 (October 1983): 1111-1115.

        The remarks of U.S. Senator, Spark Matsunaga (Democrat-
        Hawaii) on the federal role in research, treatment, and
        prevention of alcoholism. Part of his remarks are about
        employee assistance programs (EAPs) in industry and gov-
        ernment. Author biographical information. 1 photograph.
        8 footnotes.

4.063   "The Navy Fights Alcoholism." Alcohol Health and Re-
        search World (Fall 1973): 9-11.

        The U.S. Navy Alcohol Abuse Control Program (AACP) was
        established in 1971. There are five rehabilitation
        centers: Long Beach and San Diego , California; Norfolk,
        Virginia; Great Lakes, Illinois; and Jacksonville, Flor-
        ida. The U.S. Comptroller General estimates that alco-
        holism costs the Navy about $45 million annually in mil-
        itary manpower losses, excluding other costs. 3 photo-
        graphs.

4.064   "New Jersey Enacts Alcoholism Coverage." Labor-Manage-
        ment Alcoholism Journal 7 (September-October 1977): 30.

        Text of a statute mandating insurance coverage for treat-
        ing alcoholism in New Jersey.

4.065   New Jersey State Department of Health. "New Jersey Plan
        for the Prevention and Treatment of Alcoholism, 1976-77."
        Government Reports Announcements and Index 76 (December
        24, 1976): 76. NTIS HRP-0012095/6GA.

        Portions of this report deal with alcohol, unemployment,
        and occupational programs. 1 appendix.

4.066   "New Program Helps Alcoholics Find Jobs." Labor-Manage-
        ment Alcoholism Journal 8 (September-October 1978): 61.

        The Employment Program for Recovered Alcoholics (EPRA)
        in New York City began operations in June 1978. The New
        York State Department of Mental Hygiene, and the New
        York City Bureau of Alcoholism Services, provided fund-
        ing for the program.

4.067   "NIAAA's Occupational Programs Branch: Meeting the Chal-
        lenge." Alcohol Health and Research World (Fall 1973):
        6-8.

        Describes the work of occupational program consultants
        (OPCs)--men and women employed by the Occupational

Programs Branch of the National Institute on Alcohol
Abuse and Alcoholism (NIAAA). Their task is to market
employee alcoholism programs (EAPs) throughout the U.S.
Private business and government--state and local--is
the market. Prudential Insurance in Newark, New Jersey
is educating its employees about alcoholism. In Iowa,
the Iowa Institute of Public Affairs is doing similar
work. 3 photographs.

4.068   O'Connell, Michael. "Alcohol Abuse in the Public Ser-
        vice." Civil Service Review 50 (September 1977): 3-4,
        6-8 and 10-13.

        Alcohol abuse in the Canadian public service. Much of
        this article is an interview with Dr. F.H. Hicks. He
        deals with occupational health matters in the public
        service. This article contends that Canadians consume,
        on a per capita basis, more alcohol than do Americans,
        Britons or Russians. 6 photographs.

4.069   Opinion Research Corp. "Executives' Knowledge, Atti-
        tudes and Behavior Regarding Alcoholism and Alcohol
        Abuse. Study II." Government Reports Announcements
        and Index 76 (March 19, 1976): 21. NTIS PB-248 696/
        7GA.

        This report is a follow-up to a survey conducted in Jan-
        uary 1972. This and the previous survey were carried
        out by the Opinion Research Corp. of Princeton, New Jer-
        sey. Both reports were done for the National Institute
        on Alcohol Abuse and Alcoholism (NIAAA). Over 500 busi-
        ness executives took part in an interview survey. The
        executives were from banking, transportation, life in-
        surance, and other areas of business. This report, like
        the 1972 report, is made up mostly of statistical infor-
        mation. Abstract.

4.070   Orvis, Bruce R., David J. Armor, Christine E. Williams,
        Andrea J. Barras and Donna S. Schwarzbach. "Effective-
        ness and Cost of Alcohol Rehabilitation in the United
        States Air Force." Government Reports Announcements and
        Index 82 (July 16, 1982): 2954-2955. NTIS AD-A112 787/7.

        Comments on the U.S. Air Force alcohol rehabilitation
        program and remarks on its effectiveness. Then talks
        about a cost analysis of the program. One of the conclu-
        sions of the researchers is that less intensive and more
        intensive treatment interventions are about equal in ef-
        fectiveness. The researchers also found that clients im-
        proved substantially after treatment. Abstract. 1 fig-
        ure. 31 tables. 7 appendices. 27 references.

4.071   Palmer, P.V. "The Air Canada Programme for Rehabilita-
        tion of the Alcoholic Employee/Pilot." Aviation, Space
        and Environmental Medicine 54 (July 1983): 592-594.

The Air Canada employee alcoholism program (EAP) dates back to the early 1960s. The program emphasizes early detection and peer pressure. Three case histories are used in this article. Author biographical information. Abstract.

4.072   Parker, Philip H. "Washington State's Employee Alcohol- ism Program." Public Personnel Management 2 (May-June 1973): 212-215.

The state of Washington established, in January 1973, an employee alcoholism program (EAP) in the Department of Personnel. This article covers: the state's posi- tion, the responsibility of supervisors, employee rights and responsibilities, labor-management cooperation, and job performance. Author biographical information.

4.073   Pearce, Theodore. "Occupational Alcoholism Programs in France and Great Britain." Labor-Management Alcoholism Journal 6 (March-April 1977): 28-30.

Alcoholism in France was first designated an illness in 1930. The High Commission on Alcoholism is the French equivalent of the NIAAA (National Institute on Alcohol Abuse and Alcoholism) and was created in 1954. Former French Premier Mendes-France is credited with efforts to curb alcoholism in that country. In Britain, in Jan- uary 1976, the British National Council on Alcoholism formed the Working Party on Alcohol and Work. A report was issued on January 5, 1977. One of the findings: al- coholism costs British industry about $700 million annu- ally. Author biographical information.

4.074   Phillips, Donald A. "Alcoholism and Productivity." Civil Service Journal 13 (July-September 1972): 25-27.

The role of the U.S. Federal Civil Service Commission in dealing with alcoholism. The commission, for example, sponsored, in November 1967, a conference on work and problem drinking. Also, the commission cooperated with the General Accounting Office (GAO) in a study of the cost savings to the government of employee alcoholism programs (EAPs). The guidelines of Civil Service Commis- sion employee alcoholism programs are given. Author biographical information. 1 illustration.

4.075   Polich, J. Michael. "Epidemiology of Alcohol Abuse in Military and Civilian Populations." American Journal of Public Health 71 (1981): 1125-1132.

Men in the U.S. Army, Navy, and Air Force were compared with civilian populations in order to study alcohol abuse. The demographic data of military personnel was used to account for greater alcohol abuse in the mili- tary than among civilians. Abstract. 5 tables. 40 references. Author biographical information.

4.076 Polich, J. Michael and Bruce R. Orvis. "Alcohol Prob-
       lems: Patterns and Prevalence in the U.S. Air Force."
       Government Reports Announcements and Index 80 (January
       18, 1980): 196. NTIS AD-A074 740/2.

       A report prepared for the U.S. Air Force. The air force
       wanted a cost-benefit study of its alcohol abuse pro-
       gram. Military and civilian behavior were compared.
       The Rand Corp. researchers visited thirteen air force
       bases. A random sample of over 3000 active-duty air
       force personnel were surveyed. 65 tables. 9 figures.
       8 appendices. 85 references. Abstract.

4.077 Pool, Wayford C. "Los Angeles County Occupational
       Health Services Employee Alcoholism Program: A Perfor-
       mance Report for 1975." Government Reports Announce-
       ments and Index 79 (August 31, 1979): 44. NTIS PB-295
       746/2GA.

       The three major parts of this report concern: a de-
       scription of the employee alcohol program (EAP), in-
       cluding history, structure, functions, and flow of cli-
       ents through the program; funding; and accomplishments
       and problems. Over 80% of the clients had some college
       education. The program was established on January 15,
       1969. Abstract. 8 tables. 2 figures. 9 appendices.
       19 references.

4.078 "Postal Service Keeps Up with PAR." Labor-Management
       Alcoholism Newsletter 2 (September-October 1972): 1-16.

       Expansion of the Program for Alcoholic Recovery (PAR)
       throughout the U.S. Postal Service. The postal service
       has more than 700,000 employees and an annual budget of
       $10 billion. A PAR pilot model was established in San
       Fancisco in 1968. 1 photograph. 4 exhibits.

4.079 Pursch, Joseph A. "From Quonset Hut to Naval Hospital:
       The Story of an Alcoholism Rehabilitation Service."
       Journal of Studies on Alcohol 37 (1976): 1655-1665.

       Historical account of the first alcoholism treatment pro-
       gram in the U.S. Navy. Group counseling, Alcoholics
       Anonymous (AA), psychodrama, and recreational psychother-
       apy are treatment vehicles used at the Long Beach, Cali-
       fornia Alcohol Rehabilitation Service (ARS). Abstract.
       Author biographical information. 4 footnotes. 2 refer-
       ences.

4.080 "Railroad Programs Surveyed." Labor-Management Alcohol-
       ism Journal 6 (March-April 1977): 26-27.

       Reports on a Federal Railroad Administration (FRA) survey

of alcoholism and drug abuse counseling programs. Interviews with program directors and labor officials, as
well as anonymous questionnaires, were used to obtain
information. Name and address where to write for additional information is included.

4.081   Regan, Riley W. "The Role of Federal, State, Local, and
Voluntary Sectors in Expanding Health Insurance Coverage
for Alcoholism." Alcohol Health and Research World 5
Summer 1981): 22-26.

Some of the associations, agencies, and committees discussed are: Group Health Association of America, Inc.;
the Alcohol, Drug Abuse, and Mental Health Administration (ADAMHA); the Senate Alcoholism and Drug Abuse Subcommittee; the National Institute on Alcohol Abuse and
Alocoholism (NIAAA); the National Association of State
Alcoholism and Drug Abuse Directors (NASADAD); the National Association of Insurance Commissiones (NAIC);
the Joint Commission on Accreditation of Hospitals
(JCAH); and the Blue Cross/Blue Shield Service Benefit
Plan. Author biographical information. 2 illustrations.

4.082   Regional Health Planning Council of the North Central
Texas Council of Governments. "Proposed 1975 North Central Texas Regional Plan for the Prevention and Treatment of Alcohol Abuse and Alcoholism: A Summary." Government Reports Announcements and Index 77 (October 28,
1977): 58-59. NTIS HRP-0003767/1GA.

Tabular data includes information about occupational alcoholism programs (OAPs).

4.083   Reid, Angus and Neena Chappell. Overview of Alcohol/Drug
Programs in Canada. Ottawa: National Planning Committee
on Training of the Federal Provincial Working Group on
Alcohol Problems, 1978.

Covers two major areas: the social history of alcohol
and drug programming in Canada, and federal and provincial jurisdictions associated with alcohol and drug programs. There are separate sections for each of the Canadian provinces and territories. This publication is part
of a series of publications on alcohol problems in Canada. 8 tables. 10 figures.

4.084   Russell, Julia C. and Audie W. Davis. "Alcohol Rehabilitation of Airline Pilots." Government Reports Announcements and Index 86 (April 11, 1986): 31-32. NTIS AD-A
163 076/3/GAR.

Elaborates on the success--85% success rate since 1976--
of an alcoholism treatment program for airline pilots.

Success is attributed to cooperation of the pilots'
union, airline companies, and the Federal Aviation Administration (FAA). The records of nearly 600 pilots
were analyzed. Author biographical information. Abstract. 4 figures. 1 table. 11 references.

4.085   Sanders, Robert Tracy. "Alcoholism in the Navy: A
        Cost Study." Government Reports Announcements and In-
        dex 75 (July 11, 1975): 19. NTIS AD-A009 910/1GA.

        A master's thesis awarded to the author by the Naval
        Postgraduate School, Monterey, California. The four
        main areas dealt with in this thesis are: the history
        of alcohol control, program factors, alcohol-related
        navy expenses, and the navy's investment in the alcohol-
        ism prevention program. Author biographical information.
        Abstract. 2 appendices. 31 references. 80 footnotes.

4.086   Schuckit, Marc A. "Alcohol Problems in the United
        States Armed Forces." Military Chaplain's Review (Win-
        ter 1977): 9-19.

        Concentrates on three issues: epidemiology, possible
        subtypes of alcoholism in the naval services, and treat-
        ment and prevention issues. This article is based pri-
        marily on data about alcohol problems in the U.S. Navy.
        Author biographical information. 21 footnotes. 2 ta-
        bles.

4.087   Schuckit, Marc A. and E.K. Eric Gunderson. "The Asso-
        ciation between Alcoholism and Job Type in the U.S. Na-
        vy." Quarterly Journal of Studies on Alcohol 35 (1974):
        577-585.

        In this study, it was learned that there were nine jobs
        in the U.S. Navy with a high prevalence of alcoholism,
        and nine with a low prevalence. High prevalence was as-
        sociated mostly with nontechnical jobs. Low prevalence
        was associated mostly with skilled jobs requiring more
        education. Data for this study included psychiatric
        case files from the Navy Medical Neuropsychiatric Re-
        search Unit in San Diego, California. Author biographi-
        cal information. Abstract. 2 tables. 4 footnotes. 15
        references.

4.088   Schuckit, Marc A. and E.K. Eric Gunderson. "Deaths
        among Young Alcoholics in the U.S. Naval Service."
        Quarterly Journal of Studies on Alcohol 35 (1974): 856-
        862.

        In a study of deaths among young navy and marine corps
        alcoholics, it was discovered that the major cause of
        death was due to self-inflicted wounds. Author biograph-
        ical information. Abstract. 2 tables. 18 references.

4.089   Schuckit, Marc A. and E.K. Eric Gunderson. "The Evalua-
        tion of Naval Alcohol Rehabilitation Programs: Problems
        and Suggestions." Government Reports Announcements and
        Index 78 (August 18, 1978): 70. NTIS AD-A054 366/0GA.

        This paper was presented at the National Conference on
        Evaluation in Alcohol, Drug Abuse, and Mental Health
        Programs, Washington, D.C., April 1-4, 1974. Author
        biographical information. 31 references. 1 footnote.
        Abstract.

4.090   Shoemaker, Gary L. "Analysis of Specific Alcohol Risk
        Characteristics of Participants in the United States Air
        Force Supervisor Alcohol Abuse Education Program." Dis-
        sertation Abstracts International 44: 1698A. ED.D.
        dissertation, George Washington University, 1983. Order
        No. DA8324490.

        United States Air Force members--606 officers and en-
        listed members--from thirteen installations were studied.
        The reason for the study was to identify individuals
        with significant risk of alcohol abuse. Increased family
        interaction was found to be an indicator of lower risk of
        alcohol abuse.

4.091   Silsby, Harry D., Calvin Neptune, David J. Kruzich and
        Helen D. Gouin. "Establishment of the First US Army Al-
        coholism Residential Treatment Facility in the Continen-
        tal United States." Military Medicine 148 (January
        1983): 21-23.

        The first U.S. Army alcoholism residential treatment fa-
        cility, on the mainland U.S., began operation at William
        Beaumont Army Medical Center in El Paso, Texas in Novem-
        ber 1980. This article is about: the historical back-
        ground, mission and staffing, treatment issues, treatment
        programs, and profile of first-year admissions. Author
        biographical information. 1 table. 4 references.

4.092   Solomon, J. "Alcoholism and Work." Government Reports
        Announcements and Index 85 (March 15, 1985): 51. NTIS
        HRP-0906095/5/GAR.

        This publication was prepared by the Arizona Center for
        Occupational Safety and Health in Tucson, Arizona for the
        Bureau of Health Professions, Hyattsville, Maryland.
        More than 5000 major U.S. companies deal with employee
        alcoholism by means of employee assistance programs
        (EAPs). Abstract. 2 tables. 127 references.

4.093   South Central Connecticut Regional Mental Health Plan-
        ning Council. "Regional Alcoholism Plan for South Cen-
        tral Connecticut." Government Reports Announcements and
        Index 77 (May 13, 1977): 76. NTIS HRP-0012127/7GA.

Includes data about industrial and business alcoholism programs. Abstract.

4.094   Southeast Arkansas Economic Development District. "Southeast Arkansas District Plan for the Prevention, Treatment, and Control of Alcohol Abuse and Alcoholism." Government Reports Announcements and Index 76 (June 25, 1976): 45. NTIS HRP-0004551/8GA.

Contains information about industry and alcoholism.

4.095   Swint, J. Michael and David R. Lairson. "Economic Evaluation of Occupation-Based Programs: Conflicting Criteria and the Case for Government Subsidy." Journal of Studies on Alcohol 46 (1985): 157-160.

Compares, in terms of economic criteria, occupation-based programs with public rehabilitation programs. Recommends that government, via subsidies or tax credits, give employers incentive to institute quality programs. Private and public programs could then be evaluated more consistently. Author biographical information. Abstract. 3 figures. 9 references.

4.096   Swint, J. Michael and David R. Lairson. "Employee Assistance Programs: Incentives for Increasing State and Local Support." Alcohol Health and Research World 8 (Winter 1983-1984): 35-39.

Government--federal, state, and local--can encourage establishment of employee assistance programs (EAPs) through incentives such as monetary subsidies or tax credits. Author biographical information. 3 figures. 1 table. 7 references.

4.097   Tappan, J.R. "Here's to Grog!" Naval War College Review 26 (May-June 1974): 87-94.

Numerous statistics are used in this account of alcohol use and abuse in the U.S. Navy. 2 tables. 5 footnotes. 1 photograph. Author biographical information.

4.098   "Tax Credit Available for Hiring Alcoholics." Labor-Management Alcoholism Journal 10 (May-June 1981): 245.

The Targeted Jobs Tax Credit Program, of the U.S. Department of Labor, gives all private employers an opportunity to receive a tax credit for hiring hard-to-place workers. Alcoholics are frequently found in the seven target groups from which employers can choose workers.

4.099   Texas Commission on Alcoholism. "Texas State Plan for the Prevention, Treatment and Control of Alcohol Abuse

and Alcoholism: 1975." <u>Government Reports Announce-</u>
<u>ments and Index</u> 76 (October 15, 1976):   54.   NTIS HRP-
0006894/0GA.

Has information about occupational alcoholism programs
(OAPs).

4.100   Texas Commission on Alcoholism.   "Texas State Plan for
the Prevention, Treatment and Control of Alcohol Abuse
and Alcoholism, 1976." <u>Government Reports Annoncements</u>
<u>and Index</u> 77 (October 28, 1977):   71.   NTIS HRP-0015020/
1GA.

This publication includes information about occupational alcoholism.   33 exhibits.

4.101   Trice, Harrison M. and Janice M. Beyer.   "Differential
Use of an Alcoholism Policy in Federal Organizations by
Skill Level of Employees."   Chapter in <u>Alcoholism and</u>
<u>Its Treatment in Industry</u>, edited by Carl J. Schramm,
44-68.   Baltimore, MD: Johns Hopkins University Press,
1977.

The sample for this research were seventy-one, federal,
civil service organizations in the northeastern U.S.
The organizations were nonmilitary and were located in
the Boston, Philadelphia, and New York regions.   Over
600 supervisory level employees participated in the investigation.   Both high status and low status alcoholics
were studied.   6 footnotes.   4 tables.   32 references.

4.102   Trice, Harrison M., Janice M. Beyer and Cynthia Coppess.
"Sowing Seeds of Change: How Work Organizations in New
York State Responded to Occupational Program Consul-
tants." <u>Journal of Drug Issues</u> 11 (1981):   311-336.

Summarizes a Cornell University evaluation of occupational program consultants (OPCs) in New York State.
The National Institute on Alcohol Abuse and Alcoholism
(NIAAA) in 1972 funded occupational programming at the
state level.   The Cornell evaluation took three years.
Role ambiguity and role conflict characterized the role
of occupational program consultant.   Author biographical information.   Abstract.   3 tables.   5 notes.   50
references.

4.103   Trice, Harrison M., Janice M. Beyer and Richard E.
Hunt.   "Evaluating Implementation of a Job-Based Alcoholism Policy." <u>Journal of Studies on Alcohol</u> 39
(1978):   448-465.

An evaluation of the U.S. Civil Service Commission alcoholism policy.   Abstract.   Author biographical information.   1 table.   7 footnotes.   28 references.

4.104   "U.S. Coast Guard Announces Formal Alcoholism Policy."
        Labor-Management Alcoholism Journal 10 (January-Feb-
        ruary 1981):   163-164.

        An eight-point alcoholism policy announced by the U.S.
        Coast Guard.   This article includes the text of the
        policy.   The policy was proposed by the National Mar-
        itime Union (NMU).

4.105   "Volunteers Head Chicago Task Force on Employee Alco-
        holism Programs."   Labor-Management Alcoholism Journal
        6 (September-October 1976):   20-21 and 24-28.

        Profiles the members of the National Council on Alco-
        holism (NCA) steering committee on employee alcoholism
        programs (EAPs).   The members are: Alan S. Boyd, Wil-
        liam A. Lee, Morgan F. McDonnell, James J. McDonough,
        Patrick L. O'Malley, Michael Tenenbaum, Robert Johnston,
        and Louis F. Peick.   8 photographs.

4.106   Walters, Lynford S., III.   "A Contest Without a Loser:
        The Development of the Navy's Alcohol Rehabilitation
        Program."   Government Reports Announcements and Index
        82 (January 15, 1982):   252.   NTIS AD-A104 599/6.

        A master's thesis received by the author at the Naval
        Postgraduate School in Monterey, California.   The the-
        sis describes the development of the navy's alcohol
        rehabilitation program between 1965 and 1980.   Ab-
        stract.   Author biographical information.   2 appendi-
        ces.   4 figures.   21 references.

4.107   Weiss, Richard M.   "The Role of the Federal Government."
        Chapter in Dealing with Alcoholism in the Workplace, 52-
        59.   New York, NY: Conference Board, Inc., 1980.

        Covers federal support for alcoholism programs, govern-
        ment assistance and program development, government as-
        sistance and program structure, and government assis-
        tance and program processes and outcomes.   The Alcohol-
        ism Rehabilitation Act of 1968 marked the beginning of
        federal legislative efforts to deal with alcoholism.
        The Rehabilitation Act of 1973 viewed alcoholics as
        handicapped individuals.   This was an attempt to pro-
        hibit discrimination against alcoholics seeking employ-
        ment and to prevent the unjust dismissal of alcoholics.
        5 tables.

4.108   West Central Arkansas Planning and Development District.
        "West Central Arkansas Alcohol Abuse and Alcoholism
        Plan."   Government Reports Announcements and Index 76
        (March 19, 1976):   39.   NTIS HRP-0004345/5GA.

        Has information about business, industry, and occupa-
        tional services.   13 tables.   1 figure.

4.109   Whitney, Wheelock. "Employee Alcoholism Programs: Who
        Should Pay?" Labor-Management Alcoholism Journal 11
        (July-August 1981):   20-21.

        The election of Ronald Reagan as President, federal bud-
        get cuts, and occupational alcoholism programming is
        discussed.   The value to various segments of society of
        employee alcoholism programs (EAPs) is emphasized.   The
        value is reflected in both economic and noneconomic
        terms.   Author biographical information.

4.110   "Wisconsin Law Requires Alcoholism Coverage in Group
        Policies." Labor-Management Alcoholism Newsletter 2
        (September-October 1972):   22.

        On September 8, 1972, Wisconsin was the first state to
        pass a law requiring all group health insurance policies
        to cover alcoholism treatment.

4.111   "World's Largest Employer Installs Alcoholism Program."
        Labor-Management Alcoholism Newsletter 2 (July-August
        1972):   1-13 and 16-17.

        Development of an employee alcoholism program (EAP) at
        the U.S. Civil Service Commission.   2 photographs.

4.112   Yardley, Michael. "What Shall We Do with the Drunken
        Soldier?" New Statesman 102 (October 2, 1981):   15-16.

        A former lieutenant in the British army talks about sol-
        diers and alcoholism.   Author biographical information.
        2 photographs.

4.113   Zuska, Joseph J. "Beginnings of the Navy Program." Al-
        coholism: Clinical and Experimental Research 2 (October
        1978):   352-357.

        A first-person account of the development of an alcohol-
        ism treatment program in the U.S. Navy.   Many problems
        were encountered during the evolution of the program,
        including denial of drinking problems, resistance to
        treatment by individuals with alcohol abuse problems,
        and hostility by alcoholics and others towards rehabili-
        tation staff.   Author biographical information.

5

Specific Occupations

5.001 "Alcohol-Dependent Doctors." British Medical Journal 2
(August 11, 1979): 351.

Alcoholic doctors in Scotland, England, and Wales. Com-
pares treatment of British doctors with doctors in the
U.S. and Canada. Suggests that treatment programs in
North America are considerably better than in Britain.
Comments on the rehabilitation of alcoholic doctors in
New York State. 11 references.

5.002 "The Alcoholic Doctor in Need of Help." Medical Opinion 5 (December 1976): 8-11.

Interview with a recovered alcoholic doctor. The doctor, while an alcoholic, tried to commit suicide three
times. He was helped by Alcoholics Anonymous (AA), after which he had no desire for alcohol. 1 illustration.

5.003 "Alcoholism among the Medical Profession." Lancet 2
(December 2, 1978): 1215.

Reports on a symposium on alcohol abuse by doctors. The
symposium was held in January 1977. It was organized by
the Medical Council on Alcoholism and the Society for
the Study of Addiction.

5.004 Archer, Janet. "Alcoholism and Alienation among Blue
Collar Workers: Test of a Causal Theory." Dissertation
Abstracts International 42: 1339A. Ph.D. dissertation,
Johns Hopkins University, 1981. Order No. DA8120007.

One hundred and sixty male blue-collar workers were the
sample for this research. Eighty of the workers were
alcoholics; eighty were nonalcoholics. Of the four hypotheses tested, only one was supported by data--that
alcoholics experience disappointed life expectations
more frequently than do nonalcoholics.

5.005 "At Risk." Drug Merchandising 64 (February 1983): 31.

Autobiographical account of a pharmacist whose alcoholism was treated with assistance from the Manitoba Pharmacist at Risk program. 1 photograph.

5.006   Ayres, Perry R. "The Physician Alcoholic: ARCH to Recovery." Ohio State Medical Journal 73 (1977): 737-
739.

Elaborates on ARCH (Acceptance, Recognition, Confrontation, Hope)--principles and attitudes essential in the
treatment of alcoholic patients, including alcoholic
physicians. Author biographical information. 7 references.

5.007   Bates, Richard C. "The Alcoholic Attorney: What to Do?"
New York State Bar Journal 56 (January 1984): 22-24.

A doctor, with the aid of a case history, describes sev-
en things to bear in mind for the attorney who wants to
help a colleague who is an alcoholic. 1 illustration.

5.008   Bednarek, Robert J. and H. Joe Featherston. "A Program
for Hospital Employees: Analysis of First Year's Results." Labor-Management Alcoholism Journal 10 (September-October 1980): 70-83.

St. Benedict's Hospital in Ogden, Utah is sponsored by
the Order of Sisters of St. Benedict. This article comments on the hospital's alcoholism and chemical dependency treatment program after the first year of results.
1 photograph. 2 footnotes. 2 figures. 1 table. 22
references.

5.009   Bissell, LeClair and Paul W. Haberman. "Appendix D:
20 Questions Developed by California Lawyers for Their
Colleagues." in Alcoholism in the Professions, by
LeClair Bissell and Paul W. Haberman, 206-207. New
York, NY: Oxford University Press, Inc., 1984.

Criteria for detecting alcoholism in the legal profession.

5.010   Bissell, LeClair and Robert W. Jones. "The Alcoholic
Physician: A Survey." American Journal of Psychiatry
133 (October 1976): 1142-1146.

Alcoholic American and Canadian male physicians were the
sample for this research. The subjects were located
primarily through International Doctors in AA, a chapter
of Alcoholics Anonymous (AA). The subjects were administered a fifty-part questionnaire during 1968-1970.
Ninety-eight questionnaires were usable. About half of
the sample had also had problems with drugs. Abstract.
Author biographical information. 5 tables. 23 references.

5.011   Bissell, LeClair, Klaus Lambrecht and Ross A. von
        Wiegand. "The Alcoholic Hospital Employee." _Nursing
        Outlook_ 21 (November 1973):   708-711.

        An alcoholism program was established in 1968 at Roose-
        velt Hospital in New York. The department of medicine
        and department of psychiatry established the program.
        Supervisors from nursing, engineering, radiology, and
        other departments have referred staff for treatment to
        the program. Author biographical information.

5.012   Bissell, LeClair and Al J. Mooney. "The Special Prob-
        lem of the Alcoholic Physician." _Maryland State Medi-
        cal Journal_ 25 (March 1976):   79-80.

        The special problem of the alcoholic physician relates
        primarily to his prestigious position and his high de-
        gree of autonomy over his professional and personal
        life. This contributes to denial, on his part, that he
        has a drinking problem. A late diagnosis and inade-
        quate treatment often lead to a complicated clinical
        course. Author biographical information.

5.013   Blacklaws, Allan F. "One Company's Experience." Chap-
        ter in _Alcohol Problems in Employment_, edited by Brian
        D. Hore and Martin A. Plant, 134-143. London: Croom
        Helm Ltd., 1981.

        Describes how Scottish and Newcastle Breweries Ltd.
        helps its alcoholic workers. Scottish and Newcastle
        has approximately 27,000 employees. This chapter in-
        cludes an outline in point form of the company's policy
        on drinking problems at work. Also included are exam-
        ples of employees with drinking problems. The efforts
        to help employees at Scottish and Newcastle have trade
        union support.

5.014   Blose, Irwin L. "Confronting the Alcoholic Employee."
        AORN Journal 25 (May 1977):   1159-1160, 1162-1163 and
        1166.

        How the nursing supervisor can help the alcoholic nurse
        recognize her drinking problem and take constructive
        action to overcome the alcoholism. Includes a fictional
        dialogue between a nursing supervisor and an alcoholic
        nurse, illustrating constructive confrontation. Author
        biographical information. 10 references.

5.015   Boroson, Warren. "How Your Career Can Affect Your
        Drinking." _Money_ 5 (January 1976):   46-48 and 50.

        The views of three people regarding the amount of alco-
        hol a person has to consume to be an alcoholic: Paul A.
        Sherman, Director, Special Programs, International Tele-
        phone and Telegraph (ITT); Dr. Frank A. Seixas, Medical

Director, National Council on Alcoholism (NCA); and Dr. Morris E. Chafetz, former Director, National Institute on Alcohol Abuse and Alcoholism (NIAAA). Also goes into drinking and specific occupations, particularly at the management level. Employee alcoholism programs (EAPs) are also examined. 1 illustration. 1 photograph.

5.016   "Bottle and Throttle." Flying 112 (August 1985): 72-74.

Daytime and nighttime airplane accidents in which alcohol is involved.

5.017   Canfield, Mary. "Alcohol Dependency: Spotting the Tell-Tale Signs at Work." Occupational Health 33 (April 1981): 186-190.

Five case studies are used to illustrate how to spot alcohol dependency at a work environment associated with the brewing industry. Includes the names and addresses of seven facilities in Britain for the treatment of alcoholism. 1 photograph.

5.018   Casswell, Sally and Alistair Gordon. "Drinking and Occupational Status in New Zealand Men." Journal of Studies on Alcohol 45 (1984): 144-148.

Bartenders, lawyers, surveyors, and cooks were some of the occupational groups studied in this research into drinking and occupational status of thousands of New Zealand men. Social class and cirrhosis mortality were two important variables studied. The sample was questioned during 1978-1979. Author biographical information. Abstract. 3 tables. 2 figures. 17 references.

5.019   Chapman, Stu. "'I Am a Reformed Alcoholic, and I Am a Doctor.'" Legal Aspects of Medical Practice 6 (November 1978): 47-49.

An account of a New York doctor who struggled with his drinking problem for over twenty years and overcame it. Abstract. Author biographical information. 2 photographs.

5.020   Chazin, Michael. "Alcohol on the Job: A $15 Billion Hangover." Inland Printer-American Lithographer 177 (June 1976): 38-41.

Alcoholism in American industry and the printing industry in particular. Reasons why industry is hesitant to admit it has alcoholic workers. Advice on how to set up an employee alcoholism treatment program. Emphasizes nine things not to do when dealing with alcoholism. 1 illustration. 1 table. 1 chart.

5.021   Clinger, Robert D.   "Help for the Alcoholic Physician
        in Ohio." _Alcoholism: Clinical and Experimental Re-
        search_ 1 (April 1977): 139-141.

        The Ohio State Medical Association's Physician Effec-
        tiveness Program. This program began providing assis-
        tance on July 1, 1975 to physicians with alcohol and
        other problems. The voluntary program operates on six
        general principles. Problems with the program are de-
        scribed. Author biographical information.

5.022   Cocciarelli, Susan. "Alcoholism: Academics, Academe."
        _Journal of the College and University Personnel Asso-
        ciation_ 36 (Winter 1985): 1-8.

        An article which consists of two main parts. In part
        one, recovering, Michigan State University faculty mem-
        bers talk about those characteristics of the academic
        environment that may precipitate alcoholism. In part
        two, academic administrators discuss their role in
        helping faculty recover from alcoholism. Author bio-
        graphical information. 5 references.

5.023   Coller, Jerome E. "The Maryland Physician Rehabilita-
        tion Committee Program." _Maryland State Medical Jour-
        nal_ 29 (October 1980): 36-39.

        Explains the beginnings of and rationale for the Com-
        mittee on Physicians Rehabilitation in Maryland. This
        committee was appointed in September 1977 and was sub-
        sequently divided into five subcommittees. Prior to
        1977, the Commission on Medical Discipline (CMD) dealt
        with impaired physicians. The CMD could revoke a phy-
        sician's license. Author biographical information. 2
        tables.

5.024   Collins, Richard L. "Inflight Drunks: Teetering on the
        Brink." _Flying_ 112 (August 1985): 74-75.

        Negative effect of alcohol consumption on "flying a
        plane" in a SimuFlite Lear 55 simulator. 1 illustra-
        tion.

5.025   Conrad, Barnaby. "Genius and Intemperance." _Horizon_
        23 (December 1980): 33-40.

        Drinking habits of American fiction writers. Some of
        the writers discussed: Edgar Allan Poe, Mark Twain,
        Ambrose Bierce, Sinclair Lewis, Ernest Hemingway, Thomas
        Wolfe, William Faulkner, and Ring Lardner. Author bio-
        graphical information. 15 photographs.

5.026   Conwell, H.R. "Alcoholism: A Behavioural Disorder in
        General Aviation." _Aviation, Space and Environmental
        Medicine_ 54 (July 1983): 599-600.

In the U.S. between 1965 and 1975 there were over 400
general aviation accidents associated with alcohol.
This constituted 8% of the total number of general aviation accidents for that time period. How to recog-
nize, prevent, and alleviate alcoholism is covered.
Author biographical information. Abstract. 8 references.

5.027   Cook, Robert. "Cirrhosis in Doctors." Lancet 1 (January 20, 1979): 156.

Seeks clarification about the claim that liver cirrhosis among doctors is much more prevalent than among the
general population.

5.028   Cosper, Ronald and Florence Hughes. "So-Called Heavy
Drinking Occupations: Two Empirical Tests." Journal
of Studies on Alcohol 43 (1982): 110-118.

Compares drinking by U.S. military officers, most of
whom were in the navy, and journalists from Ottawa, Ontario. Comparison groups with which the military officers and journalists were compared included the general
American population and Canadian university professors
and chartered accountants. The officers and journalists drank more than their comparison groups. Author
biographical information. Abstract. 1 table. 12 references.

5.029   Cramer, Jerome. "The Alcoholics on Your Staff: How to
Find Them, How to Help Them, and Why You'll Profit from
Doing Both." American School Board Journal 164 (August
1977): 49-52.

Information about the treatment of alcoholics employed
by the Milwaukee, Wisconsin school board. This school
board first adopted an employee alcoholism policy in
1973. The alcoholics are treated at the De Paul Rehabilitation Hospital. Also described is a similar program at the Bedford Central School District in Mount
Kisco, New York. Author biographical information. 1
illustration.

5.030   Davies, John B. "Drinking and Alcohol-Related Problems
in Five Industries." Chapter in Alcohol Problems in Employment, edited by Brian D. Hore and Martin A. Plant,
38-60. London: Croom Helm Ltd., 1981.

Reports on alcohol-related problems in Clydeside, an industrial area near Glasgow, Scotland. Funds for the
study of alcohol use by industrial workers were appro-
priated in May 1977. One thousand and thirty workers
were sampled out of a total work force of 27,700. A
shipyard, vehicle manufacturer, and brewery were three
employers who participated in the study. 4 tables. 3

notes.

5.031   de Fuentes, Nanette. "A Study of Implementation and
         Evaluation of an Aerospace Employee Assistance Program."
         Dissertation Abstracts International 47: 2209B. Ph.D.
         dissertation, California School of Professional Psychol-
         ogy, Los Angeles, 1986. Order No. DA8616488.

         This research, with the aid of a review of records and
         interviews, involved over 700 people. The research
         yielded, in addition to other things, information on:
         client demographics, gender and ethnic patterns, client
         and supervisor profiles and satisfaction rates, and
         ideas for improving the employee assistance program
         (EAP).

5.032   Dean, G., R. MacLennan, H. McLoughlin and E. Shelley.
         "Causes of Death of Blue-Collar Workers at a Dublin
         Brewery, 1954-1973." British Journal of Cancer 40
         (October 1979): 581-589.

         Researchers concluded that there was a significantly in-
         creased risk of death from cancer of the rectum, and
         from diabetes mellitus, for brewery workers in Dublin,
         Ireland who consumed large amounts of beer. The same
         workers, however, did not have an increased risk of
         death from other types of cancer. Author biographical
         information. Abstract. 7 tables. 9 references.

5.033   Denenberg, Tia Schneider and R.V. Denenberg. "Hourly
         Rules." in Alcohol and Drugs: Issues in the Workplace,
         by Tia Schneider Denenberg and R.V. Denenberg, 107-108.
         Washington, DC: Bureau of National Affairs, Inc., 1983.

         Prohibition of alcohol consumption hours before report-
         ing for duty by employees in the airline industry.

5.034   Denenberg, Tia Schneider and R.V. Denenberg. "Suspicion
         of Impairment Rules." in Alcohol and Drugs: Issues in
         the Workplace, by Tia Schneider Denenberg and R.V. Denen-
         berg, 108. Washington, DC: Bureau of National Affairs,
         Inc., 1983.

         A possible alternative to the hourly rule for employees,
         who have to report for work alcoholically unimpaired. It
         is mandatory in the airline industry for certain employ-
         ees not to consume alcoholic beverages a set number of
         hours before reporting for work.

5.035   "A Disease Called Alcoholism." Medical Opinion 5 (De-
         cember 1976): 6-7.

         Many doctors still view alcoholism as a "bad habit,"
         rather than as an illness. Treating the alcoholic doc-
         tor is an especially difficult task. Colleagues are

hesitant about helping the alcoholic doctor until they have no other choice.

5.036   Dishlacoff, Leon. "The Drinking Cop." Police Chief 43 (January 1976): 32, 34, 36 and 39.

Symptoms and characteristics of alcoholism and program approaches to treatment. Author biographical information. 1 photograph.

5.037   Donaldson, Scott. "The Crisis of Fitzgerald's 'CRACK-UP.'" Twentieth Century Literature 26 (Summer 1980): 171-188.

Alcohol in the life of author, F. Scott Fitzgerald. 66 notes.

5.038   Donovan, Bruce E. "The Brown University Program: Alcoholism Focus." Chapter in Employee Assistance Programs in Higher Education: Alcohol, Mental Health and Professional Development Programming for Faculty and Staff, edited by Richard W. Thoreson and Elizabeth P. Hosokawa, 195-199. Springfield, IL: Charles C. Thomas, Publisher, 1984.

Focuses on the adaptation of existing programs to Brown University, the emphasis and openness accorded alcohol problems, and the reaching of troubled faculty. This program is available to faculty, staff, and students. This paper was presented at a Conference on Employee Assistance Programs in Higher Education held during August 3-6, 1980.

5.039   "The Drinking Doctor." Human Behavior 6 (March 1977): 31-32.

Reports on research by LeClair Bissell, a medical doctor, and Robert W. Jones, a professor of sociology. They interviewed ninety-eight doctors who are recovered alcoholics. The researchers found that the medical profession was more tolerant of the formerly alcoholic physicians than was the general public. Many doctors stated their alcoholism did not harm their patients.

5.040   Dunne, Joseph A. "Evaluating the New York City Police Department Counseling Unit." Chapter in Alcoholism and Its Treatment in Industry, edited by Carl J. Schramm, 91-108. Baltimore, MD: Johns Hopkins University Press, 1977.

Begins by discussing the development of the New York City Police Counseling Unit then talks about the alcoholism treatment program and its impact on organizational attitudes and structure. A table gives a statistical

analysis of the counseling program for the years 1966-
1974.   2 figures.   1 table.   14 references.

5.041   "Duren's New Pitch: Look Out for Booze."   _Newsweek_
101 (June 20, 1983):   13.

Ryne Duren, former star pitcher for the New York Yan-
kees, was an alcoholic who drank up to two dozen vodka
martinis a night.   He spent time in a mental institu-
tion and also threatened to jump off a bridge.   He overcame his alcoholism and works for Heitzinger and Asso-
ciates, a firm that helps athletes deal with drinking
and drug problems.   2 photographs.

5.042   "Editorial."   _Journal of Tropical Medicine and Hygiene_
79 (January 1976):   1.

Views alcoholism in the medical profession as a serious
problem.   4 references.

5.043   Edwards, Griffith.   "The Alcoholic Doctor: A Case of
Neglect."   _Lancet_ 2 (December 27, 1975):   1297-1298.

How doctors can deal with the problem of alcoholic colleagues.   Author biographical information.   2 references.

5.044   Elliott, Barbara and Etta Wiliams.   "An Employee Assistance Program."   _American Journal of Nursing_ 82 (1982):
586-587.

The employee assistance program (EAP) at Baptist Memorial Hospital in Kansas City, Missouri provides assistance to employees with alcohol or drug problems.   This
article also has information about help for alcohol and
drug abuse by nurses in Alabama, California, New Jersey,
North Carolina, and Wisconsin.   National organizations,
including addresses, are listed separately.   Author biographical information.

5.045   Fichter, Joseph H.   "Alcohol Addiction: Priests and Prel-
ates."   _America_ 137 (October 22, 1977):   258-260.

Draws parallels between priests and bishops and employees
and employers in industry.   Describes how bishops react
to their own alcohol problems, and gives reasons for
their reactions.   The National Clergy Council on Alcoholism has a program for alcoholic church personnel.   Author
biographical information.

5.046   "Florida Bar Fights Substance Abuse."   _Association Man-
agement_ 37 (December 1985):   16.

How the Florida Bar Association helps lawyers who have
alcohol and drug abuse problems.

5.047   Glatt, M.M. "Alcoholism among Doctors." Lancet 2 (August 10, 1974): 342-343.

Contends, with the aid of statistics, that doctors more frequently abuse alcohol than other drugs.

5.048   Glatt, M.M. "Alcoholism an Occupational Hazard for Doctors." Journal of Alcoholism 11 (Autumn 1976): 85-91.

Attempts to determine the extent of alcoholism among doctors and attempts to explain why certain doctors drink excessively. Also gives reasons why a "conspiracy of silence" often exists, within the medical profession, regarding alcoholic doctors. Self-help groups are examined and the need for prevention is stressed. Author biographical information. 15 references.

5.049   Glatt, M.M. "Characteristics and Prognosis of Alcoholic Doctors." British Medical Journal 1 (February 19, 1977): 507.

Discusses undergraduate and graduate factors involved in alcoholism among doctors. Hard work, frustrations, and great responsibilities contribute to physician alcoholism. Prognosis for improvement and recovery is seen as excellent. 3 references.

5.050   Godard, Jacques. "Alcohol and Occupation." Chapter in Alcohol Problems in Employment, edited by Brian D. Hore and Martin A. Plant, 105-117. London: Croom Helm Ltd., 1981.

Alcoholism and the workplace in a French context. Relates absenteeism, morbidity, industrial accidents, premature aging and premature death, and social problems to alcohol abuse. 1 table.

5.051   Gold, Todd. "Sid Caesar's New Grasp on Life." Saturday Evening Post 258 (January-February 1986): 64-65, 110 and 112.

The alcoholism of comedian, Sid Caesar. 2 photographs.

5.052   Gualtieri, Antony C., Joseph P. Cosentino and Jerome S. Becker. "The California Experience with a Diversion Program for Impaired Physicians." Journal of the American Medical Association 249 (January 14, 1983): 226-229.

In California, the Board of Medical Quality Assurance finances a treatment program for impaired physicians, including those who abuse alcohol. These physicians, by agreeing to receive help from the program, can likely avoid medical board discipline. A nondisciplinary

approach gives impaired physicians more incentive to
seek treatment because legal restrictions against the
physicians' licenses are avoided. Author biographical
information. Abstract. 4 tables. 11 references.

5.053   Haffenden, John. "Drink as Disease: John Berryman."
        Partisan Review 44 (1977): 565-583.

        Alcoholism of poet, John Berryman.

5.054   Hamill, Pete. "A Memoir of the Drinking Life." New
        York 8 (January 13, 1975): 45-48.

        Autobiographical account about the alcoholism of writ-
        er, Pete Hamill. 1 photograph.

5.055   Harper, C.R. "Airline Pilot Alcoholism: One Airline's
        Experience." Aviation, Space and Environmental Medi-
        cine 54 (July 1983): 590-591.

        Early identification of alcoholics is a cornerstone of
        the alcoholic rehabilitation program at United Airlines.
        The flight surgeon, flight manager, and union represen-
        tative regularly monitor the alcoholic employee's con-
        dition. Liver function tests and spot-checks of blood
        alcohol levels are used. Author biographical informa-
        tion. Abstract.

5.056   Harris, Jimmy Dale. "An Employee Alcoholism Program
        for Public Education." Dissertation Abstracts Interna-
        tional 37: 1328A. Ph.D. dissertation, University of
        Idaho, 1976. Order No. DA7619895.

        A systems approach was used to construct an alcoholism
        training model to be used by public school administra-
        tors for the purpose of dealing with alcohol abusing,
        public school employees.

5.057   Hingson, Ralph, Thomas Mangione and Jane Barrett. "Job
        Characteristics and Drinking Practices in the Boston
        Metropolitan Area." Journal of Studies on Alcohol 42
        (1981): 725-738.

        Thousands of people in the Boston metropolitan area were
        interviewed between November 1977 and July 1978 regard-
        ing alcohol consumption. The researchers were interest-
        ed in occupational differences in drinking practices. A
        wide spectrum of white collar and blue collar individ-
        uals took part in this study. Job stress and boredom
        were found to be related to drinking. Author biographi-
        cal information. Abstract. 4 tables. 17 references.

5.058   Holden, Constance. "Alcoholism: On-the-Job Referrals
        Mean Early Detection, Treatment." Science 179 (January
        26, 1973): 363-365, 413 and 415.

How government and industry rehabilitate alcoholic em-
ployees. The treatment program at the New York Transit
Authority is discussed at length. Programs at Merrill
Lynch, Pierce, Fenner and Smith, and at General Motors
(GM) are mentioned.

5.059   Hopkins, Jay. "A Sober Review: The Stone-Cold Sober
Truth." _Flying_ 112 (August 1985): 78 and 83.

The remarks of Jay Hopkins, Manager of Instructional Design of the SimuFlite Lear 55 simulator. Hopkins comments on the alcoholic intoxication of J. Mac McClellan
and Richard L. Collins, editors of _Flying_. McClellan
and Collins consumed alcohol then "flew" in the simulator at the Dallas-Fort Worth Airport. 1 illustration.

5.060   "Is Alcohol Abuse a Staff Problem?" _Health Care_ 24
(March 19, 1982): 18.

Spokespersons for five Canadian hospitals comment on al-
cohol abuse by hospital staff: Ralph Moore (General
Hospital Health Sciences Centre, St. John's, Newfound-
land); Gudmundur Myrdal (Seven Oaks General Hospital,
Winnipeg, Manitoba); Carey Robinson (St. Catharines
General Hospital, St. Catharines, Ontario); Royce Gill
(Regina General Hospital, Regina, Saskatchewan); and
Bernard Martin-Smith (Royal Columbian Hospital, New
Westminster, B.C.). 2 photographs.

5.061   Isenberg, Susan K. "Maintaining the Alcoholism Empha-
sis: A Consortium Model." Chapter in _Employee Assis-
tance Programs in Higher Education: Alcohol, Mental
Health and Professional Development Programming for
Faculty and Staff_, edited by Richard W. Thoreson and
Elizabeth P. Hosokawa, 209-218. Springfield, IL:
Charles C. Thomas, Publisher, 1984.

Five key topics: historical background, program revi-
talization efforts, pros and cons of a high self-referral rate, early identification of alcohol drug-related
problems, and barriers to supervisory referrals. This
paper is a revised version of a presentation at a Conference on Employee Assistance Programs in Higher Education held during August 3-6, 1980. 2 tables.

5.062   Isler, Charlotte. "The Alcoholic Nurse: What We Try
to Deny." _RN_ 41 (July 1978): 48-55.

Contends there are 40,000 alcoholic nurses in the U.S.
Dr. LeClair Bissell, Chief, Smithers Alcoholism Treatment and Training Center in New York, is quoted throughout this article. Dr. Bissell is a recovered alcoholic.
Author biographical information. 2 photographs.

5.063   Jackson, George, Lazaro Diaz and Geraldine Wallman.

"An Employee Alcoholism Program for Nurses and Social Workers." Labor-Management Alcoholism Journal 9 (November-December 1979): 115-122.

The Mount Sinai Medical Center in New York began its employee assistance program (EAP) in January 1978. The program is available to all employees, including nurses and social workers. The New York Chapter of the National Association of Social Workers prepared a manual entitled "Alcoholism among Social Workers: Approaching a Colleague with a Drinking Problem." Author biographical information. 1 figure. 23 references.

5.064   Jackson, George W. "Employee Alcoholism Programs in Hospitals." Alcohol Health and Research World 3 (Spring 1979): 18-21.

The advantages of an employee alcoholism program (EAP) at the Mount Sinai Medical Center in New York, and the difficulties encountered in establishing the program. Author biographical information. 2 illustrations. 1 chart. 3 references.

5.065   Jackson, George W. and Lazaro Diaz. "The Development and Implementation of Employee Assistance Programs in Hospital Settings." Chapter in Social Work Treatment of Alcohol Problems, edited by David Cook, Christine Fewell and John Riolo, 143-149. New Brunswick, NJ: Rutgers Center of Alcohol Studies, 1983.

Although there are in the U.S. over 7100 hospitals and medical centers, only 10% of non-federal, short-term, general hospitals offer treatment for employee alcoholism. Three hundred and one New York State hospitals were surveyed and seventy-nine responded. Of the respondents, 8.5% had a written policy for employee alcoholism. The Mount Sinai Medical Center employee assistance program (EAP) is described. 12 references.

5.066   Jervey, Gay. "Is the Advertising World a Mecca for 'Demon Rum'?" Advertising Age (February 7, 1983): M4-M5 and M40.

The alcoholism of two admen, Richard Fischer and Robert McDonald. Also discusses how two ad agencies, Young and Rubicam and N.W. Ayer, deal with their alcoholic employees. An inset section talks about alcohol and younger advertising people. Author biographical information. 2 sketches.

5.067   John, Harrison. "Alcohol and the Impaired Physician." Alcohol Health and Research World 3 (Winter 1978): 2-8.

As of June 1978, twenty-six states had programs for

impaired physicians: Arizona, California, Delaware,
Georgia, Illinois, Indiana, Kansas, Kentucky, Maryland,
Massachusetts, Michigan, Minnesota, Mississippi, Nebraska, New Jersey, North Carolina, Ohio, Oklahoma,
Pennsylvania, Rhode Island, South Carolina, Tennessee,
Texas, Utah, Washington, and Wisconsin. However, International Doctors in Alcoholics Anonymous (IDAA) has
existed since 1947. The U.S. Navy has treated alcoholic naval doctors since 1972 at the Alcoholism Rehabilitation Service in Long Beach, California. 2 illustrations. 15 references.

5.068   Johnson, Harvey L. An Exploration Study of Deviance in
the Athabasca Oil Sands Area. Edmonton: Alberta Oil
Sands Environmental Research Program, 1979.

This study of social deviance in "boom towns" of northern Alberta includes a look at alcohol abuse. The communities are: Fort McMurray, Anzac, and Fort MacKay.
These communities are associated with rapid natural resource development. They are characterized by mushroom-
ing economic activity. An influx of workers creates
population growth. Alcohol abuse and related problems
become virtually indigenous to the communities.

5.069   Kazin, Alfred. "'The Giant Killer:' Drink and the American Writer." Commentary 61 (March 1976): 44-50.

A number of American writers and their drinking behavior
is discussed, including Scott Fitzgerald, Ring Lardner,
John Berryman, and John O'Hara. Author biographical information.

5.070   King, Michael L. "Lawyers on the Rocks." American Bar
Association Journal 70 (March 1984): 78-83.

Autobiographical accounts of lawyers and their drinking
problems: J. Paul Molloy, Arnold Peebles, Jr., Theodore
Cohen, Paul Van Valkenburg, and John Holahan. Wayne
Ewen, a consultant in alcohol counseling in Texas, be-
lieves there are 95,000 alcoholic lawyers. 5 photographs. Author biographical information.

5.071   Klinefelter, Harry F. "Alcoholism in the Medical Profession." Maryland State Medical Journal 29 (October 1980):
49.

Two case reports about alcoholic physicians.

5.072   Kliner, Dale J., Jerry Spicer and Peggy Barnett. "Treatment Outcome of Alcoholic Physicians." Journal of Studies on Alcohol 41 (1980): 1217-1220.

Hazelden is an alcoholism treatment facility whose patients include, among other individuals, alcoholic

physicians. One year after eighty-five physicians were
discharged from Hazelden, each was sent a multiple-choice
questionnnaire. The purpose of the questionnaire was to
elicit information about the effectiveness of the treatment program. The authors conclude that treatment at
Hazelden is effective because over three-quarters of the
treated physicians were abstinent one year after discharge. Abstract. Author biographical information. 14
references.

5.073   Knapp, Sherry Lynn. "The Effect of Occupational Stress
        and Social Support on Alcohol Use and Abuse." _Disserta-
        tion Abstracts International_ 46: 3583B. Ph.D. disser-
        tation, Southern Illinois University at Carbondale,
        1985. Order No. DA8526708.

        Over 600 university employees were the sample for this
        study. A major finding of the investigation was that
        high levels of occupational stress do not lead to
        greater levels of alcohol use or alcohol abuse. Social
        support--particularly from coworkers and supervisors
        rather than from spouse, friends, and relatives--ap-
        pears to be a useful strategy for reducing work envi-
        ronment stress.

5.074   Lambuth, Lynn. "An Employee Assistance Program That
        Works." _Police Chief_ 51 (January 1984): 36-38.

        The Indiana State Police Employee Assistance Program
        assists officers or family members with alcohol, emo-
        tional or other problems. The program, which was es-
        tablished in 1978, has assisted thirty-eight people.
        Author biographical information. 2 photographs.

5.075   "The Lawyer and His Health: Alcoholism." _New York_
        State Bar Journal 56 (January 1984): 8-12.

        Remarks concerning alcoholism by a member of the New
        York State Bar Association (NYSBA) Committee on Lawyer
        Alcoholism. This member is a lawyer and former alcohol-
        ic who has not consumed alcohol since 1965. He re-
        ceived help from Alcoholics Anonymous (AA). 3 illus-
        trations.

5.076   LeBourdais, Eleanor. "Impaired Incisions." _Health_
        Care 27 (February 1985): 30-32.

        Alcohol abuse by Canadian health care providers, espe-
        cially doctors in Ontario, British Columbia, Alberta,
        and Saskatchewan. 1 photograph. Author biographical
        information.

5.077   Lerner, Svetlana. "The Alcohol-Impaired Pharmacist:
        The Profession Needs a Policy." _American Pharmacy NS_
        22 (April 1982): 6-8.

Employment, access to treatment, and confidentiality are covered. Has proposed APhA (American Pharmaceutical Association) policy statements, regarding physical or mental impairment, including by reason of alcohol abuse. Author biographical information.

5.078   Lewis, Gwynne V. and Peter Rawlinson. "Alcohol-Dependent Doctors." British Medical Journal 2 (September 1, 1979): 547.

Focuses on the circumstances of young alcohol-dependent doctors.

5.079   Lewy, Robert. "Alcoholism in House Staff Physicians: An Occupational Hazard." Journal of Occupational Medicine 28 (1986): 79-81.

The Michigan Alcoholism Screening Test, Self-Administered Version was mailed to 417 house staff physicians at the Presbyterian Hospital in New York. This hospital is part of the Columbia Presbyterian Medical Center. The response rate was 45%. Test results indicated that approximately 13% of the respondents were alcoholics. Author biographical information. 4 tables. 7 references. Abstract.

5.080   Madsen, William. "Reaching the Alcoholic Academic: An Anthropological Perspective." Chapter in Employee Assistance Programs in Higher Education: Alcohol, Mental Health and Professional Development Programming for Faculty and Staff, edited by Richard W. Thoreson and Elizabeth P. Hosokawa, 145-157. Springfield, IL: Charles C. Thomas, Publisher, 1984.

Begins with an examination of the cultural context of the university and ends with suggestions for reaching alcoholic faculty. Also talks about employee assistance programs (EAPs), and faculty drinking styles and attitudes. The author expresses concern about the great difficulty of convincing academics that alcoholism is a disease. This paper was presented at a Conference on Employee Assistance Programs in Higher Education held during August 3-6, 1980.

5.081   Malikin, David. "My Name Is Joe, and I Am an Alcoholic." Chapter in Social Disability: Alcoholism, Drug Addiction, Crime and Social Disadvantage, by David Malikin, 31-39. New York, NY: New York University Press, 1973.

A transit authority employee talks about his alcoholism.

5.082   McClellan, J. Mac. "Late Night, Bad Weather, Drunk Pilot." Flying 113 (January 1986): 20-21.

The crash of a Beechcraft Baron 58 airplane which de-
parted from Fulton County Airport near Atlanta, Georgia and whose destination was Moore County Airport in
Pinehurst, North Carolina. The pilot was an airline
pilot who was intoxicated. This article is based on
a report on the crash by the National Transportation
Safety Board (NTSB). Alcohol was not the only negative factor which contributed to the crash.

5.083 McClellan, J. Mac. "Marginal Safety: Some Distinctly
       Uneasy Moments." Flying 112 (August 1985): 76-77.

       A SimuFlite Lear 55 simulator is used to demonstrate
       why pilots should not consume alcohol and fly a plane.
       2 illustrations.

5.084 McMillen, Liz. "The Alcoholic Professor: Campus Is
       Ideal Environment for a Hidden Problem." Chronicle of
       Higher Education 31 (October 9, 1985): 1 and 26-27.

       University professors--including Bruce E. Donovan, Wal-
       ter Davis, and J. Giles Milhaven--discuss their prob-
       lem drinking. 3 photographs.

5.085 McMillen, Liz. "Guidelines to Help Chairmen Deal with
       Alcoholic Professors." Chronicle of Higher Education
       31 (October 9, 1985): 27.

       Lists and elaborates on seven guidelines university de-
       partment chairmen can use in dealing with alcoholic
       professors.

5.086 McMillen, Liz. "26 Questions to Aid in Identifying
       Symptoms of Alcoholism." Chronicle of Higher Education
       31 (October 9, 1985): 26.

       Self-diagnostic National Council on Alcoholism (NCA)
       criteria for identifying alcoholism.

5.087 Meyers, Jeffrey. "The Death of Randall Jarrell." Vir-
       ginia Quarterly Review 58 (Summer 1982): 450-467.

       An account of the life and death of poet, Randall
       Jarrell--his alcoholism and mental illness.

5.088 Middleton, Martha. "Help, Hope for the Alcoholic Law-
       yer." Bar Leader 6 (January-February 1981): 29-30.

       Organizations which assist alcoholic lawyers have been
       established coast-to-coast in the U.S. The following
       are some of the organizations: the City of New York As-
       sociation of the Bar Special Committee on Alcoholism,
       the Massachusetts Bar Association's Task Force on Alco-
       holism among Lawyers, and the State Bar of California's
       Alcohol Abuse Program. 1 illustration. 2 photographs.

5.089   Morales, Richard. "Drinking Patterns among Seasonal Ag-
        ricultural Workers, 1982." Dissertation Abstracts In-
        ternational 46: 3500A. Ph.D. dissertation, Syracuse
        University, 1985. Order No. DA8524430.

        Seasonal farmworkers in Upstate New York were the sample
        for this research. The research findings support the
        picture of a group of binge drinkers--not drunken mi-
        grants. The presence of family members lessens the ex-
        tent of alcohol consumption by these workers.

5.090   Mucha, Kathleen M. Preliminary Investigation of the
        Social Impact of the Proposed Alcan Gas Pipeline with
        Regard to Alcohol and Drug Problems. Victoria: Brit-
        ish Columbia Ministry of Health, Alcohol and Drug Com-
        mission, 1978.

        Alcohol abuse and pipeline construction work is de-
        scribed in the context of Alaska--particularly Fair-
        banks--and northern Canadian communities such as Fort
        St. John and Fort Nelson.

5.091   Mueller, John F. "The Problem Drinker on Your Payroll."
        Occupational Health Nursing 22 (May 1974): 13-15.

        Symptoms of alcoholism, on-the-job signs, and a course
        of action to deal with it. Author biographical infor-
        mation. 1 photograph. 9 references.

5.092   Murray, R.M. "An Epidemiological and Clinical Study of
        Alcoholism in the Medical Profession." in Aspects of
        Alcohol and Drug Dependence, edited by J.S. Madden, Rob-
        in Walker and W.H. Kenyon, 213-219. Kent: Pitman Med-
        ical Ltd., 1980.

        This paper begins with a look at occupational mortality
        from cirrhosis then comments on doctors who, because of
        alcoholism, lose their ability to practice medicine.
        Doctors treated for mental illness, the characteristics
        of alcoholic doctors, the consequences of alcoholism,
        and referral and treatment are also examined. This pa-
        per is based on the Proceedings of the Fourth Interna-
        tional Conference on Alcoholism and Drug Dependence,
        Liverpool, England. 2 tables. 36 references.

5.093   Murray, Robin M. "The Alcoholic Doctor." British Jour-
        nal of Hospital Medicine 18 (August 1977): 144 and 146-
        149.

        Frequency of alcoholism, characteristics of alcoholic
        doctors, consequences of alcoholism, referral and treat-
        ment, and outcome. 1 table. 2 figures. 32 references.

5.094   Murray, Robin M. "Characteristics and Prognosis of Al-
        coholic Doctors." British Medical Journal 2 (December

25, 1976): 1537-1539.

An investigation of alcoholism among British doctors. Their cirrhosis death rate--specifically for doctors in England and Wales--is several hundred percent that of the general population. All the doctors in this study had been patients at the Maudsley and Bethlem Royal Hospitals. Most of the doctors were middle-aged. Two case studies are included. Abstract. Author biographical information. 2 tables. 17 references.

5.095   Murray, Robin M. "The Medical Profession." Chapter in Alcohol Problems in Employment, edited by Brian D. Hore and Martin A. Plant, 61-76. London: Croom Helm Ltd., 1981.

Covers: the psychological health of doctors, causes of psychiatric disorders in doctors, contribution of specific conditions to doctors' increased morbidity, characteristics of alcoholic doctors, consequences of alcoholism, interspecialty differences, and referral and treatment. 3 tables. 2 figures.

5.096   "My Fight for Recovery against Alcoholism." New Zealand Nursing Journal 76 (March 1983): 6-9.

Autobiographical account of the alcoholism of a nurse in New Zealand. This nurse began drinking at the age of nineteen when she was a student nurse. That was during the 1940s. She describes her treatment for alcoholism, including the turning point and sobriety. 4 photographs.

5.097   Nathan, Peter E. "Alcoholism Prevention in the Workplace: Three Examples." Chapter in Prevention of Alcohol Abuse, edited by Peter M. Miller and Ted D. Nirenberg, 387-405. New York, NY: Plenum Press, 1984.

The first program discussed is the program for federal agencies in Atlanta, Georgia. The Center for Disease Control and the Federal Aviation Administration (FAA) are the two largest agencies in the program. The second program is Live for Life at Johnson and Johnson, the health care products company. The third program is for Casino Control Commission inspectors in New Jersey. Author biographical information. 9 references.

5.098   "New FAA Rules Require Crewmembers to Undergo Alcohol Tests on Request." Aviation Week and Space Technology 124 (January 27, 1986): 41.

As of April 9, 1986, crewmembers--pilots, flight engineers, and cabin attendants--will be required to take a blood alcohol test when asked to do so by police officers. The test is a new Federal Aviation Administration (FAA) requirement for airline crewmembers.

5.099   Newlove, Donald. <u>Those Drinking Days: Myself and Other</u>
        <u>Writers</u>. New York, NY: Horizon Press, 1981.

        Writers and alcoholism: John Berryman, William Faulkner,
        F. Scott Fitzgerald, Ernest Hemingway, Jack London, Rob-
        ert Lowell, Malcolm Lowry, J.P. Marquand, John O'Hara,
        Eugene O'Neill, Edwin Arlington Robinson, Theodore
        Roethke, Tennessee Williams, and Thomas Wolfe.

5.100   Newsom, John A. "Help for the Alcoholic Physician in
        California." <u>Alcoholism: Clinical and Experimental Re-</u>
        <u>search</u> 1 (April 1977): 135-137.

        The author is a recovering alcoholic who has a general
        practice in Laguna Beach, California. Dr. Newsom is al-
        so Medical Director, CARE Unit (Comprehensive Alcoholic
        Rehabilitative Environment), South Coast Hospital, South
        Laguna. He and a colleague established a physician's
        hot-line for doctors with alcohol and other problems.
        Newsom talks about some of the calls received on the hot-
        line. Author biographical information.

5.101   O'Hagan, J.J. "The Alcoholic Doctor." <u>New Zealand Med-</u>
        <u>ical Journal</u> 93 (March 25, 1981): 192-194.

        This paper, about alcoholic doctors in New Zealand, was
        presented at the Third Annual Conference, New Zealand
        Medical Society on Alcohol and Alcoholism, March 26,
        1980. Seven specific characteristics of alcoholic doc-
        tors are listed. Four reasons are given why the medical
        profession has difficulty dealing with alcoholic doctors.
        How the profession in New Zealand should respond to this
        problem is also discussed. Author biographical informa-
        tion. 20 references.

5.102   "The Ordeal of Robert Bauman." <u>National Review</u> 32 (Oc-
        tober 31, 1980): 1349.

        Alcoholism of Congressman, Robert Bauman.

5.103   "Physician Details Alcoholic Experience." <u>Pennsylvania</u>
        <u>Medicine</u> 82 (March 1979): 51-52.

        Autobiographical account of an alcoholic physician.

5.104   Pilcher, William W. "Drinking." in <u>The Portland Long-</u>
        <u>shoremen: A Dispersed Urban Community</u>, by William W.
        Pilcher, 93-94. New York, NY: Holt, Rinehart and Win-
        ston, Inc., 1972.

        An anthropologist describes the drinking behavior of
        longshoremen in Portland, Oregon.

5.105   Plant, Martin A. "Alcoholism and Occupation." Chapter
        in <u>Drinking Careers: Occupations, Drinking Habits, and</u>

Drinking Problems, by Martin A. Plant, 17-40. London:
Tavistock Publications Ltd., 1979.

Seamen, lawyers, domestic servants, company directors,
military personnel, the medical profession, and alcohol
production workers are discussed in relation to alcoholism. 3 tables.

5.106   Plant, Martin A. "Alcoholism and Occupation: A Review."
British Journal of Addiction 72 (1977): 309-316.

Brewery workers, seamen, army personnel, domestic servants, and company directors are some of the occupations
examined. This article also looks at studies of patients in treatment institutions, alcoholics known to
agencies, population surveys of drinking habits, and
mortality statistics. The article concludes that high
alcoholism rates appear to be associated with certain
occupations. The reasons why remain unclear. Author
biographical information. Abstract. 1 table. 39 references.

5.107   Plant, Martin A. "Occupation and Alcoholism: Cause or
Effect?: A Controlled Study of Recruits to the Drink
Trade." International Journal of the Addictions 13
(1978): 605-626.

Three hundred individuals in the Edinburgh, Scotland
area--150 brewery and distillery workers, and 150 con-
trols--were the sample for this study. Each of the subjects was interviewed and asked twelve questions. Research findings indicated the brewery and distillery
workers, relative to the control group, drank significantly more alcohol. Author biographical information.
Abstract. 4 tables. 2 figures. 1 appendix. 29 references.

5.108   Poldrugo, Flavio, Gian Battista Modonutti and Renzo
Buttolo. "Attitudes toward Alcoholism among Italian Future Teachers and Health Professionals." Drug and Alcohol Dependence 17 (May 1986): 31-36.

Attitudes toward alcoholism among Italian future teachers and health professionals was compared to comparable
data for the U.S. and Australia. Cultural patterning
strongly influences the attitudes of Italian students.
The university environment does not have very much effect
in changing these attitudes. Over 400 Italian students
took part in this research. Author biographical information. Abstract. 2 tables. 14 references.

5.109   "Portrait of Disaster." RN 41 (July 1978): 52-53.

Nancy H. is a registered nurse who came from a family of
alcoholics and who herself became an alcoholic.

1 photograph.

5.110   "Professional Misconduct." Report on Business Magazine
3 (September 1986):   72.

Lawyers and chartered accountants in British Columbia
can get help for alcoholism and other problems from Interlock.   Interlock is a counseling and referral service, serving 35,000 employees and sixty companies.
Both the Law Society of British Columbia and the B.C.
Institute of Chartered Accountants assist their employees through Interlock.

5.111   Pursch, J.A.   "Alcohol in Aviation: A Problem of Attitudes."   Aerospace Medicine 45 (1974):   318-321.

After commenting on normal American drinking customs,
this paper analyzes the problem of defining, diagnosing,
and treating alcoholism.   This is followed by three case
histories of pilots who have drinking problems.   Family,
colleagues, and even doctors often help alcoholic pilots
deny they have a problem.   This paper was presented at
the Forty-Fourth Aerospace Medical Convention, Las Ve-
gas, Nevada, May 7-10, 1973.   Author biographical information.   Abstract.   8 references.

5.112   Quigley, John L. and Arthur N. Papas.   "A Therapy Program for Hospital Employees."   Hospitals 47 (September
16, 1973):   60-63.

An alcoholism treatment program for hospital employees
was initiated in 1972 at Lawrence F. Quigley Memorial
Hospital, Soldiers' Home, Chelsea, Massachusetts.   This
article contains the contents of a brochure written for
supervisors at Lawrence F. Quigley Memorial.   The brochure serves as a guide for supervisors when they deal
with alcoholic hospital employees.   Author biographical
information.   2 photographs.   4 references.

5.113   Reiman, Tyrus.   "Pharmacists at Risk."   Drug Merchandising 64 (February 1983):   27-28.

The Pharmacist at Risk program was established in Manitoba with the assistance of the Manitoba Medical Association and the Alcoholism Foundation of Manitoba.
Pharmacist at Risk is based on the Manitoba Physician at
Risk program.   The latter was established because of a
similar physician organization in Minnesota.   Pharmacists who have or who are developing an alcohol or drug
dependency problem are offered confidential help by the
Pharmacist at Risk program.   2 photographs.

5.114   Rix, Keith J.B.   "Alcohol Problems and the Fishing Industry in North-East Scotland."   Chapter in Alcohol
Problems in Employment, edited by Brian D. Hore and

Martin A. Plant, 77-104. London: Croom Helm Ltd., 1981.

The Aberdeen (Scotland) and District Council on Alcoholism held a meeting, in 1975, with representatives from
the Royal National Mission to Deep Sea Fishermen. The
purpose of the meeting was to discuss alcoholism in the
fishing industry. Subsequent research into this matter
involved a literature search, a study of official publications and public records, and the use of psychiatric
records for northeast Scotland. 3 tables. 2 figures.
1 note.

5.115 Roberts, Kristi S. "Assessment and Case Management of
the Alcoholic." Chapter in Employee Assistance Programs
in Higher Education: Alcohol, Mental Health and Professional Development Programming for Faculty and Staff,
edited by Richard W. Thoreson and Elizabeth P. Hosokawa,
267-277. Springfield, IL: Charles C. Thomas, Publisher, 1984.

Issues in interviewing for alcoholism and sustaining the
recovery of the former alcoholic. 16 references.

5.116 Rohner, Sharon W. "Alcoholics in the Helping Professions: Helping One Another." Alcohol Health and Research World 6 (Summer 1982): 18-23.

Physicians, nurses, dentists, lawyers, social workers,
and clergy have alcoholism treatment programs. Some of
the specific programs: the Drug and Alcohol Nurses Association (DANA), the National Nurses' Society on Alcoholism (NNSA), Connecticut State Dental Associaton Alco-
hol-Drug Committee, the New Jersey State Bar Association Committee on Alcoholism, and the National Clergy
Council on Alcoholism and Related Drug Problems. 1 illustration. 1 reference.

5.117 Roman, Paul M. "Employee Alcoholism and Assistance Programs: Adapting an Innovation for College and University Faculty." Journal of Higher Education 51 (March-
April 1980): 135-149.

Employee alcoholism and assistance programs in industry
and in the academic environment, and how the academic
environment differs--in terms of staff performance evaluation and program implementation--from the industrial
setting. Author biographical information. 18 references.

5.118 Rosen, M. "Alcohol-Dependent Doctors." British Medical
Journal 2 (September 1, 1979): 547.

The Association of Anaesthetists of Great Britain and
Ireland, and the Royal College of Psychiatrists, initiated an alcoholism treatment program for alcohol-

dependent anaesthetists.

5.119   Roulston, Robert. "The Beautiful and Damned: The Alco-
        holic's Revenge." Literature and Psychology 27 (1977):
        156-163.

        Alcoholism in the life of F. Scott Fitzgerald and in
        his novel, The Beautiful and Damned. 13 notes.

5.120   Rozen, Leah. "Alcoholism--Few Agencies Offer Official
        Help." Advertising Age 51 (October 27, 1980): 3 and
        100-101.

        More than twenty, major ad agencies across the U.S. were
        surveyed regarding assistance for alcoholic employees.
        Young and Rubicam was the only company with a program
        which helps these employees. The program at Young and
        Rubicam is discussed in detail. Lists eight symptoms
        of alcoholism.

5.121   Russell, Robert D. "Problem Drinking in the Education
        Profession." Phi Delta Kappan 60 (March 1979): 506-
        509.

        Claims that thousands of educators are alcoholics and
        analyzes six case histories. Young educators, middle-
        aged educators, and administrators comprise the six
        case histories. Author biographical information.

5.122   Schnurr, Sonya E. "The Alcoholic Professional." Fam-
        ily and Community Health 2 (May 1979): 33-59.

        Autobiographical account of an alcoholic registered
        nurse. Author biographical information.

5.123   Schwartz, Francis R. and George J. Kidera. "Method for
        Rehabilitation of the Alcohol-Addicted Pilot in a Com-
        mercial Airline." Aviation, Space and Environmental
        Medicine 49 (May 1978): 729-731.

        In 1968, a program to assist alcoholic employees was
        established at the United Airlines Maintenance Operations
        Center in San Francisco, California. The program was
        based on data available from the National Council on Al-
        coholism (NCA) and involved management and union coop-
        eration. The program was extended to flight crew mem-
        bers in San Francisco in 1970. Author biographical in-
        formation. Abstract. 2 figures. 14 references.

5.124   Seaman, F. James. "Problem Drinking among American
        Railroad Workers." Chapter in Alcohol Problems in Em-
        ployment, edited by Brian D. Hore and Martin A. Plant,
        118-128. London: Croom Helm Ltd., 1981.

        Elaborates on a study of problem drinking by employees

in seven large railroads. The University Research Corp.
in Washington, D.C. carried out the study at the request
of the Federal Railroad Administration (FRA). The
study was done after a major train accident in Indio,
California on June 25, 1973. The accident involved two
Southern Pacific freight trains. 10 tables.

5.125   Serebro, Boris. "The Alcoholic Doctor." Lancet 1 (Feb-
        ruary 7, 1976): 315.

        Implications of treating the alcoholic doctor.

5.126   Spender, Natasha. "Chandler's Own Long Goodbye: A
        Memoir." Partisan Review 45 (1978): 38-65.

        Alcoholism of writer, Raymond Chandler.

5.127   Stege, Harry W. "Alcoholism and the Police Officer: Im-
        pact on Police Administrators." Police Chief 52 (March
        1986): 82-84.

        Thirty-five questions used to identify an alcoholic per-
        son. Thirteen objective symptoms of alcoholism.

5.128   Steindler, E.M. "Help for the Alcoholic Physician: A
        Seminar." Alcoholism: Clinical and Experimental Re-
        search 1 (April 1977): 129-130.

        An overview of alcoholic physicians. Author biographi-
        cal information. 6 references.

5.129   "10 Questions for Lawyers." New York State Bar Journal
        56 (January 1984): 19.

        Ten questions lawyers can answer to determine if they
        have a drinking problem. Phone numbers in eight New
        York State locations where help can be obtained for al-
        coholic lawyers. Five facts about alcoholism. 1 illus-
        tration.

5.130   "There's 100-Proof Help for Alcoholic Teachers." In-
        structor 87 (April 1978): 26 and 30.

        The employee assistance program (EAP) in Des Moines, Io-
        wa public schools.

5.131   Thomas, Caroline Bedell, Patricia B. Santora and John W.
        Shaffer. "Health of Physicians in Midlife in Relation
        to Use of Alcohol: A Prospective Study of a Cohort of
        Former Medical Students." Johns Hopkins Medical Jour-
        nal 146 (1980): 1-10.

        Data in this report is from the Precursors Study and is
        about former Johns Hopkins medical students. The re-
        port describes a number of findings, including alcohol

drinking habits in medical school, alcohol drinking habits ten years after graduation from medical school, estimated alcohol consumption in midlife, youthful personality characteristics of midlife drinking habit
groups, relationship of use of alcohol over time to
health status, and alcohol usage and cigarette smoking
as related to coronary heart disease. Author biographical information. Abstract. 6 tables. 30 references.

5.132   Thoreson, Richard W. "The Professor at Risk: Alcohol
Abuse in Academe." Journal of Higher Education 55
(January-February 1984): 56-72.

The academic environment is viewed as an ideal setting
for both scholarship and alcohol abuse. The high degree of workplace autonomy of the academic--for example, he has vaguely defined standards of performance--
contributes to an environment in which alcohol dependence can easily arise. Whereas the threat of job loss
highly motivates most alcoholics in industry to seek
treatment, job loss due to alcoholism in academe is not
as likely because of tenure. Author biographical information. 45 references.

5.133   Thoreson, Richard W., Kristi S. Roberts and Elizabeth A.
Pascoe. "The University of Missouri-Columbia Employee
Assistance Program: A Case Study of Implementation and
Change." Journal of the College and University Person-
nel Association 30 (Fall 1979): 51-62.

The beginnings of an employee assistance program (EAP)
at the University of Missouri-Columbia date back to
1973. The EAP in industry was the model for the University of Missouri-Columbia (UMC) program. The EAP is
structured to assist all university staff to deal with
a variety of problems, including alcoholism and di-
vorce. The university began marketing the EAP in December 1976. Brochures, posters, and other methods were
used. Author biographical information. Abstract. 16
footnotes.

5.134   "Two Tales of One City: The Philadelphia Police and
Fire Department Programs." Labor-Management Alcoholism
Journal 4 (January-February 1975): 1-23 and 26-29.

An employee alcoholism program (EAP) was established for
the Philadelphia Police Department on March 26, 1971.
The Philadelphia Fire Department launched its EAP on
January 11, 1974. Departmental policy for each of the
programs is quoted from internal correspondence. Sample
forms used when dealing with alcoholic employees are included. 10 photographs. 14 figures.

5.135   Unkovic, Charles M. and William R. Brown. "The Drunken

Cop."   Police Chief 45 (April 1978):   18-20.

Comments on literature about the alcoholic policeman and discusses alcoholism programs at the New York City Police Department and the Philadelphia Police Department. Author biographical information. 1 photograph. 12 references.

5.136   Valaske, Martin J.   "The Impaired Physician: What He Doesn't Know Will Hurt Him." Maryland Medical Journal 34 (June 1985):   558.

Concentrates on the aspect of denial in alcoholic physicians.

5.137   Van Raalte, Ronald C.   "Alcohol as a Problem among Officers." Police Chief 46 (February 1979):   38-39.

Fourteen questions asked, and answers given, in a survey of alcohol use by police officers. Author biographical information. 1 photograph. 4 references.

5.138   Vincent, Gary.   "'My Husband Is Being Treated for Alcoholism.'" Successful Farming 81 (October 1983):   20-23.

A series of letters between the editor of Successful Farming and a reader, Ruth Whitmore, details the reader's plight with her husband's alcoholism. 8 photographs.

5.139   Violanti, John, James Marshall and Barbara Howe. "Police Occupational Demands, Psychological Distress and the Coping Function of Alcohol." Journal of Occupational Medicine 25 (1983):   455-458.

Almost 900 questionnaires were mailed to police officers in western New York State. The response rate was 56%. Depersonalization, authoritarianism, cynicism, secrecy, deviance, and alcohol use were some of the variables measured. Author biographical information. Abstract. 2 tables. 2 figures. 27 references.

5.140   Violanti, John M., James R. Marshall and Barbara Howe. "Stress, Coping, and Alcohol Use: The Police Connection." Journal of Police Science and Administration 13 (1985):   106-110.

Five hundred police officers were the sample for this study. They were employed in twenty-one different police departments. Multiple regression and path analysis were used to analyze data obtained from a questionnaire distributed to each officer. Stress was found to have the greatest impact on alcohol use. Emotional dissonance and cynicism were also found to have an impact on alcohol use, although dramatically less than

stress. Author biographical information. 2 figures. 2
tables. 26 references.

5.141   Weiner, Jack B. "'What Shall We Do with the Drunken
        Sailor...?'" Chapter in Drinking, by Jack B. Weiner,
        94-121. New York, NY: W.W. Norton and Co., Inc.,
        1976.

        Reasons why management of alcohol abuse in the navy is
        superior to alcohol abuse management in the army and
        air force.

5.142   Weisman, Maxwell N. "The Physician and Alcoholism."
        Maryland State Medical Journal 29 (October 1980): 46-
        48.

        Physician as alcoholic and as careprovider to alcohol-
        ics.

5.143   "When a Colleague's Drinking Becomes Your Headache."
        RN 41 (July 1978): 31-34.

        Identifying and helping the alcoholic nurse in the work-
        place.

5.144   Whitman, Adele. Industrial Alcoholism Seminars. Cal-
        gary: Adele Whitman, 1976.

        Describes and evaluates seminars on industrial alcohol-
        ism in small oil companies in Calgary, Alberta.

5.145   Winter, Bill. "Alcoholic Lawyers: The Probation Op-
        tion." Bar Leader 5 (January-February 1980): 27.

        A number of states have alcoholism referral committees
        for lawyers with drinking problems: California, Colo-
        rado, Connecticut, Michigan, Minnesota, Missouri, New
        Hampshire, New York, Oklahoma, Pennsylvania, South Car-
        olina, Washington, and Wyoming.

5.146   Wood, Patricia Jean. "Evidence of Alcoholism among
        Professional Nurses: What Colleagues Report." Disser-
        tation Abstracts International 46: 2489B. Ph.D. dis-
        sertation, University of Michigan, 1985. Order No.
        DA8521014.

        Over 2200 registered nurses from five regions of the U.S.
        were surveyed via questionnaire regarding work and alco-
        holism. The questionnaire enabled the respondents to
        rate themselves and their colleagues.

5.147   Wulf, Gary W. "The Alcoholic Employee." Personnel
        Journal 52 (August 1973): 702-704 and 719.

        Why the alcoholic employee should not be fired. Success

of the alcoholism treatment program at Lutheran General
Hospital, Park Ridge, Illinois. Author biographical information. Abstract. 2 footnotes. 1 table. 6 references.

5.148   Young, A.S. Doc. "Don Newcombe: Baseball Great Wins
        Fight against Alcoholism." Ebony 31 (April 1976): 54-
        56, 58, 60 and 62.

        How Don Newcombe, former Brooklyn Dodgers pitching star,
        overcame his alcoholism. 13 photographs.

5.149   Zimering, Stanley and Marianne McCreery. "The Alcohol-
        ic Teacher: A Growing Concern of the Next Decade."
        Journal of Drug Education 8 (1978): 253-260.

        Profiles the alcoholic teacher, indicating this person
        does not fit stereotype descriptions of the drunk per-
        son. The alcoholic teacher is viewed in the context of
        the middle stage alcoholic. Headaches, intestinal dis-
        orders, tingling sensations in the hands, and high blood
        pressure are frequent complaints of the middle stage al-
        coholic. Seven suggestions for dealing with the alco-
        holic teacher are given. Author biographical informa-
        tion. Abstract. 17 references.

5.150   Zink, Muriel M. "Alcoholism: The Disease That Drains
        Hospital Resources Away." Hospital Financial Manage-
        ment 32 (August 1978): 32-33.

        First looks at alcoholism in a general way then looks
        specifically at alcoholic hospital employees. 4 refer-
        ences.

6

Women

6.001 Allan, Carole A. and D.J. Cooke. "Stressful Life Events
       and Alcohol Misuse in Women: A Critical Review." Jour-
       nal of Studies on Alcohol 46 (1985): 147-152.

       A critical review by Scottish researchers of literature
       on stressful life events and alcohol misuse in women.
       The researchers claim empirical evidence which would
       demonstrate that stressful life events cause excessive
       drinking in women is inconclusive. Author biographical
       information. Abstract. 1 table. 63 references.

6.002 Anderson, Sandra C. and Donna C. Henderson. "Working
       with Lesbian Alcoholics." Social Work 30 (November-De-
       cember 1985): 518-525.

       Centers on the following: the prevalence of alcohol
       problems, lesbian identity and experience, lesbians and
       alcohol, assessment and treatment issues, treatment ap-
       proaches, homophobia and the social worker, treatment
       settings, and recommendations. Abstract. 74 notes and
       references. Author biographical information.

6.003 Anderson, Sandra Caughran. "Patterns of Identification
       in Alcoholic Women." Dissertation Abstracts Interna-
       tional 37: 6757A. Ph.D. dissertation, Rutgers Univer-
       sity, New Brunswick, 1976. Order No. DA777197.

       The author researched sex role identification, parental
       personality characteristics, and adolescent self-per-
       ceptions in relation to alcoholic women. The alcoholic
       women were compared to biological sisters who were not
       alcoholics. The thirty alcoholic subjects studied were
       being treated for alcoholism in the eastern U.S.

6.004 Annis, Helen M. "Treatment of Alcoholic Women." Chap-
       ter in Alcoholism Treatment in Transition, edited by
       Griffith Edwards and Marcus Grant, 128-139. London:
       Croom Helm Ltd., 1980.

       Examines a comparison of male and female treatment

outcome, treatment findings of divergent outcome result-
s, methodological factors in divergent outcome results,
prognostic factors, self-identified treatment needs, and
background characteristics and precipitating causes.   2
tables. 50 notes.

6.005   Baldwin, Janice Irene. "Women in Transition: A Time
        of Potential Alcohol Abuse." Dissertation Abstracts In-
        ternational 47: 660A. Ph.D. dissertation, University
        of California, Santa Barbara, 1985. Order No. DA8609695.

        Women experiencing transition, including separation and
        divorce, represent a population at high risk for prob-
        lems with alcohol. The effectiveness of an alcohol pre-
        vention program is evaluated.

6.006   Barnes-Cochran, Judith L. "Sexual Satisfaction, Behav-
        iors and Dysfunction in Alcoholic Women." Dissertation
        Abstracts International 47: 777B. Ph.D. dissertation,
        Indiana University, 1985. Order No. DA8607402.

        Two groups of women--one, alcoholic, the other, nonalco-
        holic--were interviewed about sexual satisfaction, be-
        haviors, and dysfunction. There were thirty-six women
        in each group and each group was matched by four vari-
        ables. The alcoholic subjects had the greatest number
        of sexual problems when they drank.

6.007   Bates, Mildred Foster. "Sex Role Strain in Alcoholic
        Women." Dissertation Abstracts International 42:
        4149A. D.S.W. dissertation, Columbia University, 1981.

        Sixty women being treated for alcoholism were compared
        regarding sex roles to sixty general population women.
        Alcoholic women differed in a number of ways from the
        general population group. Alcoholic women, for example,
        experienced higher rates of depression and greater so-
        cial isolation.

6.008   Beary, M.D. and Julius Merry. "The Rise in Alcoholism
        in Women of Fertile Age." British Journal of Addiction
        81 (1986): 142.

        A graph and table are used to demonstrate the increase
        in alcoholism in women of fertile age in Britain. Au-
        thor biographical information. 1 table. 1 figure. 3
        references.

6.009   Beckman, Linda J. "Alcoholism Problems and Women: An
        Overview." Chapter in Alcoholism Problems in Women and
        Children, edited by Milton Greenblatt and Marc A.
        Schuckit, 65-96. New York, NY: Grune and Stratton,
        Inc., 1976.

This overview of alcoholism problems and women is primarily about the social and psychological aspects of
alcoholism. The overview examines only English language publications. Among the issues examined are:
why women abuse alcohol, the heterogeneity of women
alcoholics, the family background of female alcoholics,
how women alcoholics differ from men alcoholics, and
the personalities of wives of alcoholic men. 107 references.

6.010   Beckman, Linda J. "Women Alcoholics: A Review of Social and Psychological Studies." Journal of Studies on
Alcohol 36 (1975): 797-824.

Social history variables, treatment, and directions for
future research regarding women alcoholics is the topic
of this study. Social history variables include: family background; psychopathology in women alcoholics;
differences between male and female alcoholics; differences between women alcoholics; why women become alcoholics; self-concept and esteem; specific personality
traits; female sexuality, physiology, and mood; and sex
roles and role confusion. Directions for future research include low self-esteem and sex-role confusion
and need for womanliness. Author biographical information. Abstract. 109 references.

6.011   Beckman, Linda J. and Hortensia Amaro. "Personal and
Social Difficulties Faced by Women and Men Entering Alcoholism Treatment." Journal of Studies on Alcohol 47
(1986): 135-145.

One hundred and twenty-one alcoholics--sixty-seven wom-
en and fifty-four men--were the sample population for
this research. These subjects lived or worked in Ala-
meda or Kern county in California. Some of the research
tools used were: the Health Perceptions and Beliefs
Scale, the Multidimensional Health Locus of Control
Scale, the Behavioral Impairment Index, the Duncan Socioeconomic Index, the Rosenberg Self-Esteem Scale, and
the Dean Social Isolation Scale. Author biographical
information. Abstract. 3 tables. 54 references.

6.012   Beckman, Linda J. and Vickie M. Mays. "Educating Community Gatekeepers about Alcohol Abuse in Women: Changing Attitudes, Knowledge and Referral Practices." Journal of Drug Education 15 (1985): 289-309.

Compares the effectiveness of two workshops conducted
seven months apart in California. One hundred people--
most of whom were women--voluntarily attended the workshops. The workshops produced few changes in attitudes
and behavior concerning alcohol abuse in women, but did
increase the participants' knowledge about alcohol. Author biographical information. Abstract. 3 tables.

1 figure.   33 references.

6.013   Beyer, Janice M. and Harrison M. Trice. "A Retrospective
        Study of Similarities and Differences between Men and
        Women Employees in a Job-Based Alcoholism Program from
        1965-1977." Journal of Drug Issues 11 (1981):   233-262.

        The research sample for this study consisted of 377 men
        and women--179 women, 198 men.   These individuals were
        employed by a large, multidivisional company with offices
        throughout the U.S. All the subjects had been treated
        for alcoholism in the company's alcoholism program. One
        of the differences between the male and female alcoholics
        was that the women alcoholics were more willing to talk
        about their drinking than were the men. Author biograph-
        ical information. Abstract. 7 tables. 11 notes. 107
        references.

6.014   Blume, Sheila B. "Psychiatric Problems of Alcoholic Wom-
        en." Chapter in Alcoholism and Clinical Psychiatry, ed-
        ited by Joel Solomon, 179-193. New York, NY: Plenum
        Publishing Corp., 1982.

        Anxiety, depression, phobias, obsessions, and compulsions
        are psychiatric problems associated with alcoholic women.
        Casefinding, detoxification, and psychotherapy are three
        aspects of treatment of alcoholic women. 49 references.

6.015   "Business' Multibillion-Dollar Hangover." Nation's
        Business 62 (May 1974):   66.

        Based on remarks by Edward L. Johnson who administers an
        employee alcoholism treatment program at the Firestone
        Tire and Rubber Co. The program began in September
        1972. Surveys show that about half of all company em-
        ployees who are alcoholics are women. Lists seven ways
        in which the chronic alcoholic is different from other
        employees. 1 cartoon illustration.

6.016   Calobrisi, Arcangelo. "Treatment Programs for Alcoholic
        Women." Chapter in Alcoholism Problems in Women and
        Children, edited by Milton Greenblatt and Marc A.
        Schuckit, 155-162. New York, NY: Grune and Stratton,
        Inc., 1976.

        Describes and elaborates on the four stages of the pro-
        cess of female alcoholism: prodromal, acute, intermedi-
        ate, and chronic. Stresses the importance and value of
        a team approach to treatment. Physicians, recovered al-
        coholics, psychotherapy, psychopharmacology, and bio-
        feedback are some of the components recommended in a
        team approach to treatment. 47 references.

6.017   "Causes of Female Alcoholism." Intellect 105 (January
        1977):   213.

Views of Dr. Edith S. Gomberg on the causes of female
alcoholism. Dr. Gomberg is Professor of Social Work
at the University of Michigan.

6.018   Clarke, Sandra K. "Self-Esteem in Men and Women Alcoholics." Quarterly Journal of Studies on Alcohol 35
(1974): 1380-1381.

Forty alcoholics--twenty white men and twenty white wom-
en--were the subjects in this study of self-esteem and
alcoholism. Most of the subjects were outpatients at
the Health Department Alcoholism Clinic in Akron, Ohio.
The Q-Sort Method was used to study self-esteem. Author biographical information. Abstract. 10 references.

6.019   Cohen, Sidney. "Alcoholism and Women." Chapter in The
Alcoholism Problems: Selected Issues, by Sidney Cohen,
118-123. New York, NY: Haworth Press, Inc., 1983.

Fifteen questions and answers are used to cover the
topic of alcoholism and women. 6 references.

6.020   Corneil, Wayne. "Alcoholism Treatment Programs for Female Workers." Canadian Journal of Public Health 69
(September-October 1978): 368-370.

Compares the alcohol abuse of women who work to men who
work and are problem drinkers. Makes reference to the
role differences of men and women in work and non-work
contexts. Author biographical information. 16 references.

6.021   Corrigan, Eileen M. "Alcoholic Women in Treatment: A
Summary of Findings." Chapter in Social Work Treatment
of Alcohol Problems, edited by David Cook, Christine
Fewell and John Riolo, 109-118. New Brunswick, NJ:
Rutgers Center of Alcohol Studies, 1983.

Three main topics make up this chapter: the etiology
of problem drinking among women, the effects of alcoholism on the women and their families, and the course of
treatment and outcome. Of the 150 women who were interviewed upon entering treatment, 116 of these were interviewed at a follow-up one year later. Questionnaires
were administered to personnel from treatment agencies.
Husbands and nonalcoholic sisters were interviewed.
Data pertaining to fourteen treatment agencies and several Alcoholics Anonymous (AA) groups was used in this
research. 2 tables. 9 references.

6.022   Corrigan, Eileen M. "Employment and Drinking Outcome."
in Alcoholic Women in Treatment, by Eileen M. Corrigan,
144-145. New York, NY: Oxford University Press, 1980.

Statistical information about employment and drinking
outcome of alcoholic women in treatment.

6.023 Corrigan, Eileen M. "Women and Problem Drinking:
Notes on Beliefs and Facts." Addictive Diseases 1
(1974): 215-222.

Reasons for drinking, pattern of drinking, differences
in the results of drinking, and treatment are areas
about women and alcohol which require further research.
Author biographical information. 37 references.

6.024 Dahlgren, Lena. "Special Problems in Female Alcoholism." British Journal of Addiction, Supplement No. 1,
70 (April 1975): 18-24.

A researcher from Stockholm, Sweden, and three other individuals, talk about special problems in female alcoholism. Author biographical information. 13 references.

6.025 Diamond, Deborah L. and Sharon C. Wilsnack. "Alcohol
Abuse among Lesbians: A Descriptive Study." Journal
of Homosexuality 4 (Winter 1978): 123-142.

Ten lesbians, residing in a U.S. midwestern city and
having a mean age of twenty-six, were heavy drinkers,
problem drinkers or alcoholics. Drinking helped increase assertiveness, aggressiveness, sexual initiative,
and self-esteem. It also increased feelings of sadness
and depression. Six case summaries are used to discuss
these subjects. Author biographical information. Abstract. 3 tables. 8 reference notes. 47 references.

6.026 Edwards, Griffith. "Women with Drinking Problems."
Chapter in The Treatment of Drinking Problems: A Guide
for the Helping Professions, by Griffith Edwards, 116-
124. London: Grant McIntyre Ltd., 1982.

Nine major topics about the alcoholic woman are examined: the alcoholic woman as an especially deviant
personality, the woman alcoholic as peculiarly untreat-
able, the male view, female drinking patterns, alcoholism and the tensions of the female role, depression,
premenstrual tension, overt sexual difficulties, and
the empty nest. 7 references.

6.027 Ferrence, Roberta G. "Prevention of Alcohol Problems
in Women." Chapter in Alcohol Problems in Women: Antecedents, Consequences, and Intervention, edited by
Sharon C. Wilsnack and Linda J. Beckman, 413-442. New
York, NY: Guilford Press, 1984.

Concentrates on five main areas: the rationale for

special approaches to prevention of alcohol problems in
women, the nature and extent of these problems, risk
factors for problem drinking (includes employment), current approaches to prevention, and additional strategies
and considerations. Author biographical information.
99 references.

6.028   Fleming, Michael. "Hostility in Recovering Alcoholic
Women Compared to Non-Alcoholic Women, and the Effect of
Psychodrama on the Former in Reducing Hostility." Dis-
sertation Abstracts International 35: 1405B-1406B.
Ph.D. dissertation, United States International Univer-
sity, 1974. Order No. DA7420516.

One hundred and ten women--eighty-two recovering alcoholic females and thirty non-alcoholic females--were the
subjects in this research. Three hypotheses were tested
and the research indicated that, after sobriety, the recovering alcoholic female exhibits more hostility than
does the non-alcoholic female. Psychodrama was found to
be effective in helping the alcoholic female make a
smoother transition to a new lifestyle.

6.029   Fraser, Judy. "The Female Alcoholic." Addictions 20
(Fall 1973): 64-80.

A comparison of male and female alcoholics with an emphasis on Canadian contexts. 5 illustrations.

6.030   Gelfand, Gloria Ann. "Life Issues as Social Determi-
nants for the Meaning of Being a Woman Alcoholic: A
Theory of Loss." Dissertation Abstracts International
46: 4452B. ED.D. dissertation, Columbia University
Teachers College, 1985. DA860204.

Six women residents of a New York State, alcoholism rehabilitation facility volunteered to take part in this
research. The subjects participated in sequential interview sessions. Employment was one of six generic
themes relating to the problem of alcoholism. The author's work contributed to knowledge which indicates
there are significant differences in male and female alcoholism.

6.031   Gomberg, Edith S. "Women, Work and Alcohol: A Disturb-
ing Trend." Supervisory Management 22 (December 1977):
16-20.

The increase in consumption of alcohol by women is one
of a number of changing social patterns. This particular pattern is related to others which include clothes,
sexualtiy, and employment. Author biographical information.

6.032   Harper, Frederick D. "Educational Level and Drinking

Behaviors among Alcoholic Women." <u>Journal of Alcohol</u>
<u>and Drug Education</u> 28 (Spring 1983):   2-5.

Two hundred and four women from across the U.S. were
the research sample for this study. The subjects were
being treated for alcoholism and were from urban, sub-
urban, rural, and small town areas. The women were
categorized into five educational levels: nine or fewer years, ten to twelve years, some college, college
degree, and some graduate school study. 2 tables. 5
references.

6.033 Hawkins, James L. "Lesbianism and Alcoholism." Chap-
       ter in <u>Alcoholism Problems in Women and Children</u>, ed-
       ited by Milton Greenblatt and Marc A. Schuckit, 137-
       153. New York, NY: Grune and Stratton, Inc., 1976.

       Features of this chapter include homosexual stereo-
       types, a sampling of the Los Angeles homosexual commu-
       nity, and information about gay-oriented alcoholism
       programs. The latter include the Alcoholism Program
       for Women (APW), the Van Ness House Program, and Alco-
       holics Together (AT). 34 references.

6.034 Hennecke, Lynne and Vernell Fox. "The Woman with Alco-
       holism." Chapter in <u>Alcoholism: A Practical Treatment</u>
       <u>Guide</u>, edited by Stanley E. Gitlow and Herbert S. Pey-
       ser, 181-191. New York, NY: Grune and Stratton, Inc.,
       1980.

       It is difficult to find, before the 1960s, studies on
       the alcoholic woman. Research conclusions have tradi-
       tionally been based on male samples and applied to wom-
       en. Physiological and treatment considerations of al-
       coholic women are examined. 21 references.

6.035 Henning, Nelson L. "Military Wives: Stress, Strain
       and Alcohol Use." <u>Government Reports Announcements and</u>
       <u>Index</u> 86 (November 21, 1986): 41. NTIS AD-A170 853/6/
       GAR.

       A self-administered questionnaire was used in this study
       of drinking behavior and life satisfaction, involving
       119 military wives experiencing long term separation
       from their husbands. 16 tables. 3 figures. 127 refer-
       ences. 2 appendices.

6.036 Hurwitz, Jacob I. and Dalpat K. Daya. "Non-Help-Seek-
       ing Wives of Employed Alcoholics: A Multilevel Inter-
       personal Profile." <u>Journal of Studies on Alcohol</u> 38
       (1977): 1730-1739.

       The subjects of study were the wives of alcoholic, blue-
       collar employees on the U.S. east coast. The women were
       interviewed and given personality tests. Personality

test scores revealed, in part, that the wives had a mas-
ochistic self-image. Abstract. Author biographical information. 1 figure. 1 table. 6 footnotes. 21 references.

6.037   James, Jane E. "Symptoms of Alcoholism in Women: A
        Preliminary Survey of A.A. Members." Journal of Studies
        on Alcohol 36 (1975): 1564-1569.

        Important differences were found in a comparative study
        of female alcoholics, when the alcoholism symptomatology
        of E.M. Jellinek was compared with that formulated by
        the author. Author biographical information. Abstract.
        1 figure. 1 chart. 5 references.

6.038   Johnson, Paula B. "Sex Differences, Women's Roles and
        Alcohol Use: Preliminary National Data." Journal of So-
        cial Issues 38, No. 2 (1982): 93-116.

        Over 2100 men and women, representing a national sample,
        were the subjects researched for this study. The pur-
        pose of the study was to compare alcohol consumption and
        alcohol-related problems for the two sexes. Divorced
        men and women, and unemployed men and women, exhibited
        the highest rates of consumption and problems. An ear-
        lier version of this paper was presented in Toronto, On-
        tario in 1978 at the American Psychological Association
        Annual Meeting. Author biographical information. Ab-
        stract. 4 tables. 3 reference notes. 26 references.

6.039   Jones, Ben Morgan and Marilyn K. Jones. "Women and Al-
        cohol: Intoxication, Metabolism, and the Menstrual Cy-
        cle." Chapter in Alcoholism Problems in Women and Chil-
        dren, edited by Milton Greenblatt and Marc A. Schuckit,
        103-136. New York, NY: Grune and Stratton, Inc., 1976.

        Describes alcohol intoxication levels, ethanol metabo-
        lism, and the relationship of intoxication levels to
        ethanol metabolism in women and men. Also describes a
        proposed model of alcoholism in women, behavioral ef-
        fects of alcohol on women and men, and the menstrual cy-
        cle and personality factors. 6 figures. 5 tables. 78
        references.

6.040   Kirkpatrick, Jean. "A Self-Help Program for Women Alco-
        holics." Alcohol Health and Research World 6 (Summer
        1982): 10-12.

        Compares Alcoholics Anonymous (AA) and Women for Sobri-
        ety (WFS). AA began in 1935, WFS in 1975. Author bio-
        graphical information. 1 illustration. 4 references.

6.041   Kleeman, Barbara and Bradley Googins. "Women Alcoholics
        in Management: Issues in Identification." Alcohol
        Health and Research World 7 (Spring 1983): 23-28.

Based on case studies of ten women managers, who obtained assistance for alcoholism from an employee assistance
program (EAP) at a northeastern U.S. company. Absenteeism, job autonomy, work impairment, drinking on the job,
and appearance are major issues covered. 1 illustration.
15 references. Author biographical information.

6.042   Kleeman, Barbara Esther. "Women Alcoholics in Manage-
        ment: Identification and Intervention in the Workplace."
        Dissertation Abstracts International 43: 1090A. ED.D.
        dissertation, Boston University School of Education,
        1982. Order No. DA8220942.

        Ten women in management, employed at a public utility,
        were interviewed. The women were contacted through the
        company's alcoholism program. The experiences of women
        alcoholics vary, depending on variables such as job lev-
        el and sex of supervisor.

6.043   Logan, Diane. "Marital Adjustment and Interaction be-
        tween Recovered Alcoholic Wives and Their Husbands."
        Dissertation Abstracts International 41: 4510A. Ph.D.
        dissertation, University of Georgia, 1980. Order No.
        DA8107927.

        Marital factors unique to alcoholic couples were inves-
        tigated by comparing the communication patterns of alco-
        holic and nonalcoholic couples. Fifty-three couples
        took part in the research. The Dyadic Adjustment Scale,
        Expression of Emotion Scale, Self-Disclosure Scale, and
        Inventory of Marital Conflict were used in the study.

6.044   Maletzky, Barry M. and James Klotter. "The Prevalence
        of Alcoholism in a Military Hospital." Military Medi-
        cine 140 (April 1975): 273-275.

        The research setting for this study was the Lyster Army
        Hospital at Fort Rucker, Alabama. Two hundred and
        eighty male and female patients, admitted to the medical-
        surgical ward during January 1973, were studied. The
        authors learned that 17.1% of the patients were alcohol-
        ics. Female alcoholics were outnumbered by male alco-
        holics three to one. Author biographical information.
        12 references.

6.045   Maroni, Judith. "Alcoholic Women: A Study of Their Re-
        covery Process." Dissertation Abstracts International
        47: 995B. D.N.Sc., Catholic University of America,
        1986.

        In this study of seventeen recovering alcoholic women,
        the author identified five phases of recovery: reacting,
        surrendering, strengthening, internalizing, and tran-
        scending. An open-ended interview method and theoreti-
        cal sampling were used.

6.046   Masi, Fidelia A.   "The Employed Woman Alcoholic: Problems, Solutions, and Outreach Strategies."   Labor-Management Alcoholism Journal 6 (May-June 1977):   39-44.

Three major topics: the employed woman today, the employed woman alcoholic and her problems, and solutions
and outreach strategies.   Author biographical information.   1 photograph.   5 footnotes.   1 figure.

6.047   Maxson, Charles Elvin.   "Alcoholism and Suicide among
Females."   Dissertation Abstracts International 42:
2034A-2035A.   Ph.D. dissertation, University of California, Los Angeles, 1981.   Order No. DA8122822.

The author worked with data pertaining to all non-homi-
cide deaths of Caucasian females in 1976, reported to
the Los Angeles County Medical Examiner-Coroner.   The
author sent questionnaries to individuals identified in
the coroner's records, for example, next-of-kin.   The
questionnaire response rate was 66%.   The theoretical
perspectives of Durkheim, Menninger, and others were
taken into account by the author.

6.048   McFadden, Kathryn Mary.   "The Social Support Systems of
Alcoholic Women: A Panel Analysis."   Dissertation Ab-
stracts International 47:   798B.   Ph.D. dissertation,
University of Nevada, Reno, 1985.   Order No. DA8608693.

The subjects of study were forty-three alcoholic women.
They were investigated regarding social support systems
and relapse drinking.   The women were administered questionnaires which measured variables such as family social support and negative life stress.

6.049   Milstead-O'Keeffe, Robin J.   "Meeting the Needs of Working Women with Alcohol Problems."   Labor-Management Alcoholism Journal 10 (September-October 1980):   50-60 and
65-69.

Discussed are: the Community Agency of Labor and Management (CALM) in Columbus and Franklin County, Ohio, Women
for Sobriety (WFS), and Employee-Managed Program on Wom-
en Employees' Recovery (EMPOWER).   1 photograph.   Author
biographical information.   5 tables.   3 exhibits.   13
footnotes.

6.050   Parker, Douglas A., Elizabeth S. Parker, Jacob A. Brody
and Ronald Schoenberg.   "Alcohol Use and Cognitve Loss
among Employed Men and Women."   American Journal of Public Health 73 (1983):   521-526.

Nearly 1400 employed men and women were the sample population for this investigation.   These individuals were
employed in the metropolitan Detroit area.   They were
interviewed for the authors by the Policy Research Corp.

The more alcohol the subjects consumed, the more their abstraction abilities decreased. Author biographical information. Abstract. 2 tables. 2 figures. 19 references.

6.051   Parks, Brenda Alfonso. "Participant Perceptions of Facilitator Effectiveness in the Navy Alcohol Safety Action Program." Dissertation Abstracts International 42: 3873A-3874A. ED.D. Florida State University, 1981. Order No. DA8203755.

In a study of male and female facilitators, in the Navy Alcohol Safety Action Program (NASAP), female facilitators were seen as highly effective much more often than were male facilitators. A total of 218 facilitators took part in this research.

6.052   Pinder, Lavada and Bernard Boyle. "Double-Jeopardy Employees." Addictions 24 (Fall 1977): 18-35.

Alcoholic women in the workplace in Canada. Differences between men and women in the same workplace are compared. Author biographical information. 5 illustrations.

6.053   Poley, Wayne, Gary Lea and Gail Vibe. "Working Women and Their Drinking Behaviour." in Alcoholism: A Treatment Manual, by Wayne Poley, Gary Lea and Gail Vibe, 59-60. New York, NY: Gardner Press, Inc., 1979.

Reasons for an increase in alcoholism among women in general and working women in particular.

6.054   Reichman, Walter, Marguerite Levy, Douglas Young, Stephen Herrington and Elaine Kamm. "Women's Occupational Alcoholism Demonstration Project." Labor-Management Alcoholism Journal 10 (May-June 1981): 209-218.

Reports on the preliminary findings of the Women's Occupational Alcoholism Demonstration Project in New York. February 1982 is the project completion date. Men and women, from four large organizations in the northeast U.S., participated in this project. The participants represented a diversity of occupations in the public and private sectors. The Alcohol Stage Index (ASI) was used to measure alcohol problems among the project subjects. Author biographical information. 7 tables.

6.055   Robinson, Sue Dobbs. "Women and Alcohol Abuse--Factors Involved in Successful Interventions." International Journal of the Addictions 19 (1984): 601-611.

Families, helping professions, and medical factors in relation to eighteen alcoholic women who sought treatment. One table is about employer responses to the women and their drinking. Author biographical information.

Abstract.   4 tables.   6 references.

6.056   Rossi, Jean J.   "Women and Alcohol Problems."   in <u>Treat-ment</u>, by Jean J. Rossi, 15-18.   Ottawa: National Plan-ning Committee on Training of the Federal Provincial Working Group on Alcohol Problems, 1978.

Talks about factors associated with women and alcohol problems.   Sex-role confusion, low self-esteem, and mar-ital problems are three factors.   This publication is part of a series of publications on alcohol problems in Canada.

6.057   Sandmaier, Marian.   "Employed Women."   Chapter in <u>The Invisible Alcoholics: Women and Alcohol Abuse in Amer-ica</u>, by Marian Sandmaier, 127-143.   New York, NY: Mc-Graw-Hill Book Co., 1980.

Two case histories illustrate working women and alcohol-ism.

6.058   Sandmaier, Marian.   "Freeing Women."   Chapter in <u>The In-visible Alcoholics: Women and Alcohol Abuse in America</u>, by Marian Sandmaier, 231-245.   New York, NY: McGraw-Hill Book Co., 1980.

Relationship between sexism and female alcoholism, and the meaning of real freedom for both sexes.

6.059   Sandmaier, Marian.   "Getting Help for a Drinking Prob-lem: A Woman's Guide."   Chapter in <u>The Invisible Alco-holics: Women and Alcohol Abuse in America</u>, by Marian Sandmaier, 246-274.   New York, NY: McGraw-Hill Book Co., 1980.

How and where women can get help for themselves or for others who are alcoholics.   Listed is information about: treatment programs, support groups, informational mate-rials on women and alcohol, local resource guides, multi-resource and referral centers, sources of specific ser-vices, activist groups and organizations, and further readings.

6.060   Sandmaier, Marian.   "The Hazards of Treatment."   Chapter in <u>The Invisible Alcoholics: Women and Alcohol Abuse in America</u>, by Marian Sandmaier, 206-230.   New York, NY: McGraw-Hill Book Co., 1980.

Obstacles to the treatment of female alcoholics are root-ed in stereotype images of femininity.   Alcoholism has been viewed as a male rather than female condition.   Wom-en have been seen as being more emotional than men and more likely to be psychologically maladjusted.

6.061   Sandmaier, Marian.   "The Making of an Alcoholic Woman."

Chapter in <u>The Invisible Alcoholics: Women and Alcohol Abuse in America</u>, by Marian Sandmaier, 82-105. New York, NY: McGraw-Hill Book Co.. 1980.

Attempts to explain why some women become alcoholics. Social and psychological factors are discussed, including the dependency theory. It was developed by William and Joan McCord.

6.062   Schlaadt, Richard G. and Peter T. Shannon. "Women and Alcohol." in <u>Drugs of Choice: Current Perspectives on Drug Use</u>, by Richard G. Schlaadt and Peter T. Shannon, Second Edition, 166-167. Englewood Cliffs, NJ: Prentice-Hall, 1986.

The marked increase in female alcoholism, differences between male and female alcoholism, alcohol and female physiology.

6.063   Schlesinger, Susana Jimenez. "Self-Esteem and Purpose in Life: A Comparative Study of Women Alcoholics." <u>Dissertation Abstracts International</u> 44: 678A. Ph.D. dissertation, Loyola University of Chicago, 1983. Order No. DA8317422.

One hundred and twenty volunteer subjects--alcoholic women, alcoholic men, nonalcoholic women, and nonalcoholic men--took part in this study. There were thirty adults in each of the four groups. The subjects were administered two tests: the Coopersmith Self-Esteem Inventory, Adult Form and the Crumbaugh-Maholick Purpose-in-Life Test, Part A.

6.064   Schneider, Philip V. "There Is a Better Way to Help Troubled Employees." <u>Office</u> 89 (May 1979): 46, 50 and 146.

Case study of a female alcoholic employed by a computer company in California, and how the company's employee assistance program (EAP) helped her with her drinking problem. Author biographical information. 1 figure.

6.065   Schuckit, Marc A. and Elizabeth R. Morrissey. "Alcoholism in Women: Some Clinical and Social Perspectives with an Emphasis on Possible Subtypes." Chapter in <u>Alcoholism Problems in Women and Children</u>, edited by Milton Greenblatt and Marc A. Schuckit, 5-35. New York, NY: Grune and Stratton, Inc., 1976.

Among the many factors associated with women alcoholics are: hormones, femininity, sex roles, family, spouse, sex, power, tension, and personality. This chapter also compares male and female alcoholics, and examines the prognosis and treatment of the woman alcoholic. 5 tables. 97 references.

6.066   Schuckit, Marc A. and George Winokur. "A Short Term Fol-
        low Up of Women Alcoholics." Diseases of the Nervous
        System 33 (1972): 672-678.

        The sample for this follow up study were female alcohol-
        ics who had been patients at two hospitals in St. Louis--
        the Renard Hospital and the Malcolm Bliss Mental Health
        Center. The patients, originally studied in 1967 and
        1968, were given a structured interview, and relatives
        were also interviewed. Nearly half the women designated
        as good outcome could resume social drinking. Author
        biographical information. 2 tables. 19 references.

6.067   Sclare, A. Balfour. "Alcohol Problems in Women." in Al-
        coholism and Drug Dependence: A Multidisciplinary Ap-
        proach, edited by J.S. Madden, Robin Walker and W.H.
        Kenyon, 181-187. New York, NY: Plenum Press, 1977.

        Alcohol problems in women in Britain, specifically in
        Scotland. This research was originally presented at the
        Third International Conference on Alcoholism and Drug De-
        pendence, Liverpool, England, April 4-9, 1976. 14 ref-
        erences.

6.068   Shore, Elsie R. "Alcohol Consumption Rates among Man-
        agers and Professionals." Journal of Studies on Alco-
        hol 46 (1985): 153-156.

        Approximately 250 men and women in managerial and profes-
        sional positions were the sample for this research. The
        research took place in a midwestern U.S. city. The sub-
        jects represented a variety of occupations, including
        law, personnel, advertising, and accounting. Married
        men were found to consume less alcohol than single, di-
        vorced or separated women. Author biographical informa-
        tion. Abstract. 2 tables. 24 references.

6.069   Silver-Hoffman, Linda Gail. "Factors Underlying the Use
        of Alcohol among Professional Women and Their Policy Im-
        plications: A Multivariate Approach." Dissertation Ab-
        stracts International 38 (1977): 3734A. Ph.D. disser-
        tation, Brandeis University, 1977. Order No. DA7725047.

        The sample for this investigation were over 1500 women
        who belonged to professional women's organizations in the
        Boston area. A questionnaire was mailed to the subjects
        and the response rate was approximately 50%. Some find-
        ings: wine and liquor were more preferable than beer,
        over 10% of the respondents were abstinent, and one re-
        spondent drank up to a pint of liquor daily.

6.070   Smart, Reginald G. "Female and Male Alcoholics in Treat-
        ment: Characteristics at Intake and Recovery Rates."
        British Journal of Addiction 74 (1979): 275-281.

Presents data for 157 female alcoholics and 157 male alcoholics treated in Ontario. Results are analyzed in
terms of: demographic characteristics, scale results at
intake--other than drinking, drinking characteristics at
intake, type and extent of treatment, outcomes at follow-
up, and factors associated with improvement. Author
biographical information. 3 tables. 19 references.

6.071   Stokes, Emma Jean. "Alcoholic Women in Treatment: Factors Associated with Patterns of Help-Seeking." Dissertation Abstracts International 39 (1978): 1111A. Ph.D.
dissertation, Brandeis University, 1977. Order No. DA-
7811010.

Seventy-two alcoholic women, entering alcoholism treatment, were interviewed regarding their help-seeking behavior. The loss of a meaningful relationship--for example, through death of spouse--precipitated problem
drinking in these women. Age, social class, marital status, and social role are discussed in relation to the
help-seekers.

6.072   Summey, Margaret. "The Role of Women in Occupational Alcoholism and the Special Needs of Alcoholic Women Employees." Labor-Management Alcoholism Journal 7 (May-June
1978): 15-20.

Points out differences between male and female alcoholics. Comments on women alcoholics in Atlanta, Georgia.
Author biographical information. 1 photograph.

6.073   Trice, Harrison M. and Janice M. Beyer. "Women Employees and Job-Based Alcoholism Programs." Journal of Drug
Issues 9 (1979): 371-385.

Begins with an examination of the key strategies in male-
oriented policies regarding job-based alcoholism programs.
This is followed by a discussion of the trend toward
equalization of male and female drinking and alcoholism.
The article then looks at the use of extant data to adapt
male-oriented programs, the differences between the male
and female work worlds, implications for job-based programs, and adapting constructive confrontation and crisis
precipitation to female employees. The article ends with
two major issues in adaptation--stressful life events and
suicide. Author biographical information. Abstract. 3
notes. 75 references.

6.074   Trice, Harrison M. and Paul M. Roman. "Opportunities and
Pressures." in Spirits and Demons at Work: Alcohol and
Other Drugs on the Job, by Harrison M. Trice and Paul M.
Roman, Second Edition, 31-32. Ithaca, NY: New York
State School of Industrial and Labor Relations Cornell
University, 1978.

Work-based opportunities and pressures for employed individuals, and the "empty-nest" phase of a housewife's
life, offer times and places for deviant drinking.

6.075   Vallee, Brian. <u>Life with Billy</u>. Toronto: Seal Books,
1986.

Alcoholism, wife abuse, employment problems, murder.
Nonfiction account about Jane Stafford, a Canadian woman
who was a victim of wife abuse by an alcoholic husband
she subsequently murdered.

6.076   Whitehead, Paul C. and Roberta G. Ferrence. "Liberated
Drinking: New Hazard for Women." <u>Addictions</u> 24 (Spring
1977): 36-53.

Alcoholic beverage consumption trends, alcohol-related
problems among women, and how to prevent further alcohol-related problems among this group. This article is
based on a paper presented in 1976 at the Twenty-Second
International Institute on the Prevention and Treatment
of Alcoholism held in Vigo, Spain. Author biographical
information. 5 photographs.

6.077   Williams, Carol N. and Lorraine V. Klerman. "Working
Women." in <u>Alcohol Problems in Women: Antecedents,
Consequences, and Intervention</u>, edited by Sharon C. Wilsnack and Linda J. Beckman, 282. New York, NY: Guilford Press, 1984.

Statistics about women and work.

6.078   Williams, Madeline. "The Under-Utilization of Industrial Alcoholism Programs for Women." <u>Labor-Management Alcoholism Journal</u> 10 (May-June 1981): 219-222.

Data from the Department of Health, Education and Welfare, the U.S. Postal Service, and the New York State
Division of Alcoholism and Alcohol Abuse indicates under-utilization of alcoholism programs by women. Sex
biases and reluctance by supervisors represent barriers
to detecting and treating female alcoholics. Concen-
trating on sex role conflicts, assertiveness, and self-
esteem is very important in effectively treating women
alcoholics. Author biographical information. 1 photograph. 13 references.

6.079   Wilsnack, Richard W., Sharon C. Wilsnack and Albert D.
Klassen. "Women's Drinking and Drinking Problems: Pat-
terns from a 1981 National Survey." <u>American Journal of
Public Health</u> 74 (1984): 1231-1238.

Data for this study was obtained by the National Opinion
Research Center. Over 900 women were interviewed. Research results were examined in relation to drinking

levels, adverse consequences of drinking, patterns of
consumption and consequences, and subgroup differences
in heavy consumption and consequences. Author biographical information. Abstract. 7 tables. 41 references.
1 appendix.

6.080   Wilsnack, Sharon C. "The Impact of Sex Roles on Women's
        Alcohol Use and Abuse." Chapter in Alcoholism Problems
        in Women and Children, edited by Milton Greenblatt and
        Marc A. Schuckit, 37-63. New York, NY: Grune and
        Stratton, Inc., 1976.

        Looks at sex roles and sex-role identity, psychological
        theories of female drinking, a study of female social
        drinking, womanliness and female alcoholism, recent evi-
        dence on drinking and sex roles, and changing sex roles
        and women's drinking. 9 footnotes. 74 references.

6.081   "Working Wives: Driven to Drink?" Science News 114
        (September 16, 1978): 197.

        Reports on research by Paula B. Johnson. Johnson did
        a study about alcohol consumption by women for the De-
        partment of Psychology at the University of California,
        Los Angeles, and for the Rand Corp. One of Johnson's
        findings was that married, employed women drink more
        heavily than women who are single and work or women who
        are housewives.

7

Counseling and Treatment

7.001   "Alcohol-Induced Brain Damage and Its Reversibility."
         Nutrition Reviews 38 (January 1980): 11-12.

         Abstinence from alcohol brings about in alcoholics im-
         provement of memory and learning ability. Motor im-
         pairment and brain volume are also partially revers-
         ible. Abstract. 7 references.

7.002   Alcoholics Anonymous. Living Sober. New York, NY:
         Alcoholics Anonymous World Services, Inc., 1975.

         Thirty-one tips from Alcoholics Anonymous (AA) on liv-
         ing sober.

7.003   "Alcoholics Anonymous as an Occupational Program Re-
         source." Labor-Management Alcoholism Journal 7 (Sep-
         tember-October 1977): 31-34.

         A panel presentation moderated by Weldon Butterworth,
         Director, Occupational Program Services, Alcoholism
         Council of Greater Los Angeles. The participants, in
         addition to a member of Alcoholics Anonymous (AA), in-
         cluded Ed Furtado (Northrup Corp.), John Newton (Union
         Oil Co.), and Jack Guest (Hughes Aircraft Corp.).

7.004   "Alcoholism Programs Needed." Labour Gazette 75 (Au-
         gust 1975): 485.

         Allan Clemens, of the Canadian Unemployment Insurance
         Commission, states the social stigma of alcoholism pre-
         vents development of employee alcoholism treatment pro-
         grams in Canadian industry.

7.005   "Alcoholism Treatment Center Designed to Look Like
         Home." Hospitals 57 (September 16, 1983): 63-64.

         Describes the Arms Acres Alcoholism Treatment Center in
         Carmel, New York. The center, designed by Schofield/
         Colgan of Nyack, New York, occupies fifty-four acres.

A few of the features of the center include a sauna, exercise room, meeting room, indoor swimming pool, chapel,
and dining room. 4 photographs.

7.006 Allen, Pat Buoye. "Integrating Art Therapy into an Alcoholism Treatment Program." American Journal of Art
Therapy 24 (August 1985): 10-12.

The author conducted art therapy for two years in a hospital as part of a short-term alcoholism treatment program. Author biographical information. 7 references.

7.007 "Anti-Alcohol Products." American Family Physician 28
(October 1983): 360.

Action by the Food and Drug Administration (FDA) to pro-
hibit sale of products that prevent intoxication.

7.008 Appelbaum, Steven H. "A Human Resources Counseling Model: The Alcoholic Employee." Personnel Administrator
27 (August 1982): 35, 37-38, 40-42 and 44.

The economic impact of employee alcohol abuse on companies is mentioned, including North American Rockwell
Corp., Gulf Oil Canada Ltd., Illinois Bell Telephone Co.,
Anaconda, American Brass Co., Canadian Pacific, Western
Electric Co., and Dow Chemical. Ten points to use as a
guideline in identifying the alcoholic employee are giv-
en. Also listed are fourteen points to bear in mind in
approaching the alcoholic employee about his drinking
problem. Author biographical information. 4 figures.
2 references.

7.009 Argeriou, Milton and Velandy Manohar. "Relative Effectiveness of Nonalcoholics and Recovered Alcoholics as
Counselors." Journal of Studies on Alcohol 39 (1978):
793-799.

Problem drinkers, participating in the Services for
Traffic Safety Project in Boston, were counseled by two
groups of counselors. One group consisted of former alcoholics; the other group did not have any alcohol problems. The recovered alcoholics were more effective as
counselors than were the counselors who did not have any
present or past drinking problems. Author biographical
information. Abstract. 2 tables. 22 references.

7.010 Austin, Donald G. "Let's Disagree Without Being Dis-
agreeable." Labor-Management Alcoholism Journal 10 (September-October 1980): 62-63.

Disagreement about treating alcoholism is evident among
many divergent groups, including Alcoholics Anonymous
(AA). Author biographical information.

7.011   Barton, Rufus Biggs, Jr. "A Case Study of Twenty-Five
        Rehabilitated Alcoholic Managers." <u>Dissertation Ab-
        stracts International</u> 35: 3206A-3207A. Ph.D. disser-
        tation, University of Arkansas, 1974. Order No. DA74-
        28133.

        The case study method and personal interviews were used
        to investigate rehabilitated alcoholic managers who were
        members of Alcoholics Anonymous (AA). The author wanted
        to test the developmental hypothesis of alcoholism.

7.012   Basker, Anne G. "A Useful Resource for a Neglected Ar-
        ea." <u>Labor-Management Alcoholism Journal</u> 10 (July-Au-
        gust 1980): 20-21.

        Stresses the value of Al-Anon Family Groups as a treat-
        ment resource for family members of alcoholics. Al-Anon
        is self-supporting, members do not pay dues, and there
        is extensive anonymity for members. Furthermore, Al-
        Anon does not accept donations from outside sources.
        Author biographical information. 2 footnotes.

7.013   Baum-Baicker, Cynthia. "Treating and Preventing Alcohol
        Abuse in the Workplace." <u>American Psychologist</u> 39 (April
        1984): 454.

        Why certain strategies to reduce alcohol abuse in the
        workplace have failed in the past, and an alternative
        strategy to use. Author biographical information. 10
        references.

7.014   Beavers, Carol Haught. "An Evaluation of the Impact of
        an Employee Assistance Program on Alcohol Abusing Employ-
        ees." <u>Dissertation Abstracts International</u> 46: 3250B.
        Ph.D. dissertation, Georgia State University, College of
        Education, 1984. Order No. DA8525625.

        One hundred and fifty-five employees who abuse alcohol
        were the subjects for this research. The employees were
        divided into a treatment group and two comparison groups.
        Two things the author was particularly interested in were
        employee behavior and health costs. Days absent, disci-
        plinary incidents, and the amount of medical benefits
        paid were other variables of interest to the author.

7.015   Becker, Natalie. "A Psychoanalytic Treatment Guide to
        Alcoholism." <u>Dissertation Abstracts International</u> 46:
        1330B. Ph.D. dissertation, Union for Experimenting Col-
        leges and Universities, 1984. Order No. DA8512131.

        Contends that psychoanalytic psychotherapy can be used
        to treat alcoholics. Case examples are discussed and
        treatment is detailed.

7.016   Bensinger, Ann and Charles F. Pilkington. "An

Alternative Method in the Treatment of Alcoholism: The
United Technologies Corporation Day Treatment Program."
Journal of Occupational Medicine 25 (1983):   300-303.

Describes the United Technologies Corp. day treatment
program for alcoholic employees. The program is available at the company's counseling center in New Britain,
Connecticut. Many alcoholics do not require lengthy
inpatient hospitalization. The day program is popular
with numerous employed alcoholics and their families.
United Technologies found that effective treatment outcome was not necessarily associated with long treatment
and high treatment costs. Author biographical information. Abstract. 11 references.

7.017   Berkowitz, Howard. "Prepayment for Alcoholism Treat-
        ment: The New Three-Party Matrix." Labor-Management
        Alcoholism Journal 6 (November-December 1976): 18-21
        and 24-29.

        An interview with Howard Berkowitz, Research and Devel-
        opment Division, Blue Cross Association, Chicago, Illi-
        nois.

7.018   Bhatia, Pritam Singh. "An Evaluation Model for Alcohol-
        ism Programs." Dissertation Abstracts International 38:
        478A. Ph.D. dissertation, Case Western Reserve Univer-
        sity, 1976. Order No. DA7711970.

        An attempt to develop a multiphasic and multilevel mod-
        el for describing the alcoholic client. The Multipha-
        sic Matrix for the Diagnosis of Alcoholism (MMDA) was
        used for this purpose.

7.019   Bingham, Marcia and Thomasine Gallagher. "Treatment for
        Alcoholic Employees." Hospital Progress 58 (April 1977):
        70-73 and 105.

        Mercy Hospital and Medical Center in Chicago has a
        twelve-point policy regarding employee alcoholism. A
        case history is used to illustrate treatment for alcohol-
        ic employees. A similar program at St. Therese Hospital
        in Waukegan, Illinois is mentioned. Author biographical
        information. 2 photographs. 1 figure.

7.020   Blackford, Charles E., III. "What Does Employee Alco-
        holism Really Cost?" Labor-Management Alcoholism Jour-
        nal 7 (May-June 1978):   22-23.

        Looks at quantifiable costs involved in employee alco-
        holism programs then talks about eight non-quantifiable
        savings associated with these programs. Workplace ac-
        cident reduction, tardiness, unpaid absence, and re-
        placement training costs are four of the eight non-quan-
        tifiable savings. Author biographical information. 1

photograph.

7.021   Blum, Terry C. and Paul M. Roman. "The Social Trans-
        formation of Alcoholism Intervention: Comparisons of
        Job Attitudes and Performance of Recovered Alcoholics
        and Non-Alcoholics." Journal of Health and Social Be-
        havior 26 (December 1985): 365-378.

        After discussing Alcoholics Anonymous (AA) and alco-
        hol-problem intervention, this paper looks at the his-
        tory of the employment of recovered alcoholics in the
        alcoholism field. Recovered alcoholics are then com-
        pared with non-alcoholics in terms of job attitudes and
        adjustment, and job performance. Author biographical
        information. Abstract. 2 tables. 8 notes. 34 refer-
        ences.

7.022   Bockar, Joyce A. "Alcohol and Alcoholism." Chapter in
        Primer for the Nonmedical Psychotherapist, by Joyce A.
        Bockar, 109-114. New York, NY: Spectrum Publications,
        Inc., 1976.

        Advice to the nonmedical psychotherapist who may have
        to deal with an alcoholic patient. The advice concerns
        alcohol as a drug, alcohol addiction, and Korsakoff's
        Psychosis.

7.023   Bonk, James Raymond. "Perceptions of Psychodynamics
        During a Transitional Period as Reported in Families
        Affected by Alcoholism." Dissertation Abstracts Inter-
        national 46: 634B. Ph.D. dissertation, University of
        Arizona, 1984. Order No. DA8504749.

        Twenty families were studied regarding a number of vari-
        ables, including family cohesion, dynamics, and family
        social functioning as these variables related to a fam-
        ily passing from a drinking to a non-drinking state.

7.024   Booz-Allen and Hamilton, Inc. "A Seminar on Marketing
        the Occupational Alcoholism Program." Government Re-
        ports Announcements and Index 76 (April 2, 1976): 18.
        NTIS PB-248 809/6GA.

        Booz-Allen and Hamilton, Inc., a Washington, D.C. man-
        agement consulting firm, prepared this publication for
        the National Institute on Alcohol Abuse and Alcoholism
        (NIAAA). The report reviews the need for the seminar,
        discusses the products of the seminar sessions, summa-
        rizes occupational alcoholism programs (OAPs) and the
        efforts of the NIAAA, talks about seminar products or-
        ganized by problem statement, and has a section on sem-
        inar products organized by functional categories. Ab-
        stract. 3 appendices.

7.025   Braunstein, William B., Barbara J. Powell, John F.

McGowan and Richard W. Thoreson. "Employment Factors
in Outpatient Recovery of Alcoholics: A Multivariate
Study." Addictive Behaviors 8 (1983): 345-351.

The subjects for this investigation were from the VA
(Veterans Administration) Medical Center in Lexington,
Kentucky. All 174 subjects had primary alcoholism and
were assigned to one of three treatment groups. Employed alcoholics, compared to unemployed alcoholics,
were associated with more positive treatment outcome.
Author biographical information. Abstract. 6 tables.
30 references.

7.026   Brewer, Colin. "Supervised Disulfiram in Alcoholism."
British Journal of Hospital Medicine 35 (February 1986):
116 and 118-119.

Disulfiram has not been widely used in treating alcoholism in Britain. This paper gives reasons why this drug
should be used. Disulfiram is said to be effective and
has low toxicity. Disulfiram should be used as only
one component of treatment. Author biographical information. Abstract. 1 table. 23 references.

7.027   Bucky, Steven F. et al. "Treatment." Chapter in The
Impact of Alcoholism, by Steven F. Bucky et al, 75-112.
Center City, MN: Hazelden, 1978.

Four ways of rehabilitating alcoholics: through Alcoholics Anonymous (AA), biofeedback, psychodrama, and power
motivation training (PMT). 1 table. 4 figures.

7.028   Calderone, John August. "Outcomes of a Cognitive Treatment Approach with Employed and Unemployed Alcohol Abusers on Measures of Self-Concept, Belief Systems, and Attitudes of Leisure." Dissertation Abstracts International 39: 4726A. Ph.D. dissertation, University of Pittsburgh, 1978. Order No. DA7902687.

Serenity West is an alcoholism treatment center located
in Erie, Pennsylvania. Sixty male and female alcohol
abusers took part in alcoholism research at Serenity
West. Research instruments used included the Personal
Beliefs Inventory, A Study of Leisure, Tennessee Self-
Concept Scale, and the Statistical Package for Social
Sciences (SPSS).

7.029   Carpenter, Thomas P. "An Expression of Gratitude." Labor-Management Alcoholism Journal 6 (November-December
1976): 22-23.

The relationship, past and present, between Alcoholics
Anonymous (AA) and employee alcoholism programs (EAPs).
Author biographical information. 1 photograph.

7.030   Cerrato, Paul L. "Can Diet Control the Urge to Drink?"
        RN 49 (July 1986): 63-64.

        The Wernicke-Korsakoff Syndrome and hypomagnesemia are
        two nutrient deficiencies to which chronic alcoholics
        are vulnerable. Diet therapy can replenish micronutri-
        ents lost through alcoholism, even though this therapy
        is not likely to cure alcoholism. Author biographical
        information. 1 illustration. Recommended reading list.

7.031   Chakerian, Armen and Joseph Schenkel. "In Support of a
        Consolidated Alcoholism Treatment Program." Newsletter
        for Research in Mental Health and Behavioral Sciences
        15 (November 1973): 37-41.

        Data for this investigation was obtained from the Vet-
        erans Administration Hospital in Albuquerque, New Mex-
        ico. The authors were interested in investigating the
        extent to which hospitalized patients were treated for
        alcohol related disease, but not for alcoholism itself.
        The authors viewed treatment for alcohol related dis-
        ease as an inefficient way of dealing with alcoholic
        patients. The authors recommend a comprehensive treat-
        ment program. Author biographical information. 4 ta-
        bles. 2 references.

7.032   Clark, William D. "Alcoholism: Blocks to Diagnosis
        and Treatment." American Journal of Medicine 71 (Au-
        gust 1981): 275-286.

        Presents a rational framework for diagnosing alcoholism
        and discusses counseling principles for effectively
        treating alcoholic patients. Author biographical infor-
        mation. Abstract. 1 table. 1 appendix. 54 refer-
        ences.

7.033   Cockram, Frank. "The Battle of the Bottle." CTM: The
        Human Element 14 (August 1982): 17-18.

        Seriousness of alcohol abuse by Canadian workers and
        what can be done to curb this abuse. Author biographi-
        cal information.

7.034   Cohen, Sidney. "Alcoholics: Can They Become Social
        Drinkers?" Chapter in The Substance Abuse Problems, by
        Sidney Cohen, 298-302. New York, NY: Haworth Press,
        Inc., 1981.

        A critique of a Rand report, "Alcoholism and Treatment,"
        published in June 1976. The report is about moderate
        drinking by former alcoholics. The critique lists four
        points of a general nature. This is followed by eight
        specific points. 10 references.

7.035   Coney, John Charles. "The Precipitating Factors in the

Use of Alcoholic Treatment Services: A Comparative
Study of Black and White Alcoholics." _Dissertation Abstracts International_ 37: 606A-607A. Ph.D. dissertation, Brandeis University, 1976. Order No. DA7616251.

Black and white alcoholics, at the Dimock Community
Health Center Alcoholism Program in Roxbury, Massachusetts, were studied by the author. A total of 123 individuals participated. Some of the variables taken
into account were: information on family composition,
prior alcoholic treatment affiliation, social problems,
and socioeconomic status.

7.036   Connelly, Eugene Joseph. "Predictions of Patient At-
        trition from an Alcohol Rehabilitation Program." _Dis-
        sertation Abstracts International_ 43: 265A-266A. Ph.D.
        dissertation, University of Minnesota, 1981. Order No.
        DA8211466.

        A Veterans Administration Medical Center was the set-
        ting for this study. One hundred and fifty-nine sub-
        jects took part in the research. Research instruments
        used included: the Dean Alienation Scale, Berger Self-
        Acceptance and Other-Acceptance Scale, and Moos Ward
        Atmosphere Scale.

7.037   Cordoba, Oscar A. "Drugs in the Management of Alcohol-
        ism." _Hospital Practice_ 18 (November 1983): 102A,
        102B, 102F and 102H.

        Examples of drugs used in the management of alcoholism
        include: benzodiazepines, haloperidol, chlordiazepoxide,
        diazepam, disulfiram. Author biographical information.
        7 references.

7.038   Costello, Raymond M. "Alcoholism Treatment and Evalua-
        tion: In Search of Methods." _International Journal of
        the Addictions_ 10 (1975): 251-275.

        Reports on fifty-eight evaluations of alcoholism treat-
        ment between 1951 and 1973. Author biographical infor-
        mation. 2 tables. 65 references.

7.039   Crawford, R.J.M. "Treatment Success in Alcoholism."
        New Zealand Medical Journal 84 (August 11, 1976): 93-
        96.

        A study of male and female alcoholics treated for alco-
        holism at the Queen Mary Hospital (QMH) in Hanmer
        Springs, New Zealand. The 313 men and women were treat-
        ed in 1971 and followed up for two years. Three reasons
        are given for treatment success, three for failure. The
        female alcoholics had a treatment success rate 13.2%
        higher than the male alcoholics. Author biographical
        information. Abstract. 5 tables. 19 references.

7.040   Creegan, Kevin Paul. "The Effect of Group Membership
        Similarity and Problem Relevance on Alcoholic Subjects'
        Perceptions of a Counselor's Expertness and Attractive-
        ness." Dissertation Abstracts International 46: 1332B.
        Ph.D. dissertation, State University of New York at Al-
        bany, 1984. Order No. DA85066406.

        Seventy-six patients, taking part in alcoholic treat-
        ment programs, were the subjects for this research.
        These subjects used the Counselor Rating Form to rate
        the counselor.

7.041   Cripe, Lloyd Irven. "MMPI Differences of Male Alcohol-
        ic Treatment Successes and Failures." Dissertation Ab-
        stracts International 35: 4165B. Ph.D. dissertation,
        University of Minnesota, 1974. Order No. DA752093.

        The author wanted to determine the predictive potential
        of the Minnesota Multiphasic Personality Inventory
        (MMPI) in alcoholism treatment. The subjects were male
        alcoholics. Eight hypotheses were examined.

7.042   Dagadakis, Zaharenia Stamatios. "Prediction as a Tool
        in Alcoholism Treatment." Dissertation Abstracts Inter-
        national 40: 2295A. Ph.D. dissertation, Washington
        State University, 1979. Order No. DA7923475.

        Investigated the feasibility of a prediction model for
        alcoholism treatment and concluded that such a model is
        feasible.

7.043   Dana, Robert Quinn. "Pretreatment Assertion Levels as
        They Relate to Treatment Outcome in an Alcohol Abusing
        Sample." Dissertation Abstracts International 46:
        956B. ED.D. dissertation, George Peabody College for
        Teachers of Vanderbilt University, 1984. Order No.
        DA8511232.

        In this investigation, twenty-two subjects took the Al-
        cohol Assertion Inventory, Short-Form; Michigan Alcohol-
        ism Screening Test (MAST); and Alcohol Consumption Re-
        cord. Three hypotheses were tested regarding pretreat-
        ment assertion levels as they relate to treatment out-
        come.

7.044   Davies, D.L. "Services for Alcoholics." Chapter in Al-
        coholism in Perspective, edited by Marcus Grant and
        Paul Gwinner, 102-112. London: Croom Helm Ltd., 1979.

        A look at present and future services for alcoholics,
        including medical, social, and detoxification services.

7.045   Denney, Douglas R. "Behavioral Approaches to the Treat-
        ment of Alcoholism." Chapter in Empirical Studies of
        Alcoholism, edited by Gerald Goldstein and Charles

Neuringer, 75-113. Cambridge, MA: Ballinger Publishing Co., 1976.

Three main behavioral approaches in the treatment of
alcoholism: aversion conditioning procedures, operant
procedures, and broad spectrum approaches. 100 references.

7.046   Desmond, Thomas Clark. "A Descriptive Study of Method
of Referral as a Predictor of Treatment Outcome among
Alcoholic Patients." Dissertation Abstracts International 41: 1907A. ED.D. dissertation, Boston University School of Education, 1980. Order No. DA8024089.

Four types of referral for treatment of alcoholics were
studied: self, physician, employer, and legal system.
Participants in the study responded to a questionnaire
and were treated at the Overlook Hospital in Summit,
New Jersey. The Initial Contact Form, Alcoholic Intake
Interview, and One Year Follow-Up Questionnaire are three
of the instruments used to collect data.

7.047   "Detoxification Therapy." American Family Physician 31
(March 1985): 269 and 272.

Describes the use of lithium by Dr. Lewis L. Judd and
Dr. Leighton Y. Huey in controlling alcoholism. The two
California medical doctors had, as voluntary subjects,
thirty-five chronic alcoholics.

7.048   Edwards, Daniel W. "The Evaluation of Troubled-Employ-
ee and Occupational Alcoholism Programs." Chapter in
Occupational Alcoholism Programs, edited by Richard L.
Williams and Gene H. Moffat, 40-135. Springfield, IL:
Charles C. Thomas, Publisher, 1975.

Most of this chapter is a review of publications about
employee alcoholism programs (EAPs). Other parts of the
chapter cover: a model for program planning and evaluation, sources of bias in alcoholism treatment research,
evaluations of treatment programs, and guidelines for
evaluating occupational programs. 8 tables. 1 figure.
61 references.

7.049   Edwards, Griffith. "Alcoholics Anonymous." Chapter in
The Treatment of Drinking Problems: A Guide for the
Helping Professions, by Griffith Edwards, 226-234. Lon-
don: Grant McIntyre Ltd., 1982.

Why therapists should know about Alcoholics Anonymous
(AA) as an option in the treatment of alcoholism. 7
references.

7.050   Elkin, Michael. "Common Pitfalls in Working with Alcoholics." in Families under the Influence: Changing

Alcoholic Patterns, by Michael Elkin, 81-84. New York,
NY: W.W. Norton and Co., Inc., 1984.

Common pitfalls in working with alcoholics are illus-
trated by referring to Games People Play, a book by
Eric Berne. Berne speaks about the "Rescue Triangle," a
pattern/game that requires at least two players. A
victim and a rescuer are the two players. This is applied to the alcoholic and the person who attempts to
help him.

7.051   Emrick, Chad D., Joel Hansen and Jeanne C. Maytag.
"Cognitive-Behavioral Treatment of Problem Drinking."
Chapter in The Addictions: Multidisciplinary Perspec-
tives and Treatments, edited by Harvey B. Milkman and
Howard J. Shaffer, 161-173. Lexington, MA: Lexington
Books, 1985.

The disease model of alcoholism cannot fully explain
alcoholism. Cognitive-behavioral theory is an alternative to viewing alcohol abuse as a disease. Many pro-
ponents of cognitive-behavioral theory are in the social
science field. Two case histories of cognitive-behavioral treatment of problem drinking are included. 39
references.

7.052   Ewing, John A., Thomas Dukes and Clark Sugg. "Physician Care of Alcoholics: A Survey in Central North
Carolina." North Carolina Medical Journal 33 (1972):
859-861.

There was a 46% response rate by physicians in Wake
County, North Carolina, when they were sent a brief
questionnaire concerning their care of alcoholics.
These physicians, in the opinion of the authors, were
the individuals to identify alcoholism at the earliest
stage possible. Author biographical information. 1
figure. 1 table. 8 references.

7.053   Faris, Don. "Cost of Treatment." in Economics and Social Costs, by Don Faris, 23. Ottawa: National Planning Committee on Training of the Federal Provincial
Working Group on Alcohol Problems, 1978.

Economics of alcoholism treatment facilities in Canada.
This publication is part of a series of publications on
alcohol problems in Canada.

7.054   Farr, Helen L.K., Patricia Gualtieri and Clarice Leslie.
"Training for Occupational Alcoholism Programmers: Instructional Objectives and Recommendations." Government Reports Announcements and Index 78 (December 22,
1978): 32. NTIS PB-285 809/OGA.

Presents the results of an evaluation of an occupational

programming project carried out, between April 1977 and March 1978, by the National Center for Alcohol Education (NCAE). Abstract. Glossary.

7.055   Felde, Robert. "Alcoholics Before and After Treatment: A Study of Self-Concept Changes." Newsletter for Research in Mental Health and Behavioral Sciences 15 (November 1973): 32-34.

This study took place at the Veterans Administration Hospital in Sheridan, Wyoming. The Tennessee Self-Concept Scale was used to assess the self-concept of the thirty-five alcoholic subjects. The treatment program consisted of group psychotherapy, clinical education, attitude therapy, manual arts, physical, educational, industrial, and occupational therapies. Author biographical information. 1 table. 2 references.

7.056   Fink, Edward B., Richard Longabaugh, Barbara M. McCrady, Robert L. Stout, Martha Beattie, Ann Ruggieri-Authelet and Dwight McNeil. "Effectiveness of Alcoholism Treatment in Partial Versus Inpatient Settings: Twenty-Four Month Outcomes." Addictive Behaviors 10 (1985): 235-248.

This research favored the partial hospital setting over the inpatient setting in the effectiveness of alcoholism treatment. Author biographical information. Abstract. 6 tables. 28 references.

7.057   Finke, Linda M. "The Effect of an Educational Program on the Role Security of Medical-Surgical Nurses towards Confronting Clients with Drinking Problems." Dissertation Abstracts International 46: 3390B-3391B. Ph.D. dissertation, Miami University, 1985. Order No. DA85-26792.

Alcoholism is associated with social consequences and financial losses, and is the fourth leading health problem in the U.S. Two groups of nurses of similar age, educational background, and work experience were compared regarding interventions by nurses with problem drinkers. Only one of the two groups of nurses had taken an alcoholism educational program. Nurses that had attended the program were more confident about confronting alcoholics about their problem behavior.

7.058   Flynn, Kevin Charles. "Psychometric Correlates of Involvement in a Six-Week Alcoholism Treatment Program." Dissertation Abstracts International 35: 1406B. Ph.D. dissertation, Fordham University, 1974. Order No. DA-7419657.

The author was interested in finding out to what degree psychometric instruments can predict an alcoholic's

involvement in a treatment program. The subjects were
inpatients at the Brooklyn Veterans Administration Hospital. The rehabilitation program consisted, in part,
of group therapy, and occupational and manual arts
therapies.

7.059   Follmann, Joseph F., Jr. "Appendix B: Employment-Centered Alcoholism Control Programs in Operation in 1975."
in Alcoholics and Business: Problems, Costs, Solutions,
by Joseph F. Follmann, Jr., 189-191. New York, NY:
AMACOM, 1976.

This appendix lists approximately 140 organizations
which in 1975 had an employment-centered alcoholism control program.

7.060   Follmann, Joseph F., Jr. "Appendix C: Sources of Help
and Guidance in Establishing an Alcoholism Control Program." in Alcoholics and Business: Problems, Costs,
Solutions, by Joseph F. Follmann, Jr., 192-211. New
York, NY: AMACOM, 1976.

A list of names and addresses of almost 400 sources of
help and guidance in establishing an alcoholism control
program.

7.061   Foote, Andrea and John C. Erfurt. "Effectiveness of
Comprehensive Employee Assistance Programs at Reaching
Alcoholics." Journal of Drug Issues 11 (1981): 217-
232.

Four main topics are discussed: theoretical differences between alcohol-focused and comprehensive programs,
identification and confrontation by people other than
supervisors, impact of overt program focus on alcoholism,
and the numbers of alcoholics within alcohol-focused versus comprehensive programs. Author biographical information. Abstract. 6 tables. 9 references.

7.062   Forrest, Gary G. "Antabuse Treatment." Chapter in Alcoholism and Substance Abuse: Strategies for Clinical
Intervention, by Thomas E. Bratter and Gary G. Forrest,
451-460. New York, NY: Free Press, 1985.

Antabuse has been used in treating alcoholism for more
than thirty years, even though this drug's specific
mechanism of action is not known. Antabuse does not
cure alcoholism and it is not addictive. After antabuse
treatment, the abstinence rate varies between 50% and
77%. 19 references.

7.063   Fort, Joel. "Treatment of Alcoholism." Chapter in Alcohol: Our Biggest Drug Problem, by Joel Fort, 120-135.
New York, NY: McGraw-Hill Book Co., 1973.

Drugs and psychotherapy in the treatment of alcoholism.

7.064   Fortin, Mary Lynch. "Detoxification, Then What?" American Journal of Nursing 80 (1980): 113-114.

The experiences of nursing students--from the University
of California, San Francisco--who participated in a pilot study, in which the students helped alcoholic patients before and after the patients left the hospital
detoxification units. 1 sketch. Author biographical
information.

7.065   Freedberg, Edmund J. and William E. Johnston. "Changes
in Drinking Behavior, Employment Status and Other Life
Areas for Employed Alcoholics Three, Six and Twelve
Months after Treatment." Journal of Drug Issues 9
(1979): 523-534.

This investigation involved 365 people who were administered the Ontario Problem Assessment Battery (OPAB),
as part of the research into their drinking behavior
and employment status. One year after treatment: 79%
had retained their jobs, 13% had been fired, and 62%
showed significant improvement in their drinking behavior. Author biographical information. Abstract. 7
tables. 20 references.

7.066   Freedberg, Edmund J. and William E. Johnston. "Effects
of Assertion Training within Context of a Multi-Modal
Alcoholism Treatment Program for Employed Alcoholics."
Psychological Reports 48 (1981): 379-386.

This work revealed the positive value of assertion
training within the context of a multi-modal alcoholism
treatment program for employed alcoholics. One hundred
and one alcoholic subjects took part in the research.
Fifty-six received assertion training, forty-five did
not. At a one-year follow-up, it was discovered that
the subjects who had received assertion training achieved
better results on four outcome measures--for example,
work performance and job retention. Author biographical
information. Abstract. 4 tables. 20 references.

7.067   Freedberg, Edmund J. and William E. Johnston. "Effects
of Various Sources of Coercion on Outcome of Treatment
of Alcoholism." Psychological Reports 43 (1978): 1271-
1278.

The sample here consisted of 123 subjects--120 males and
three females. All were severe problem drinkers. Almost all had been referred for treatment by their employers. Nine sources of coercion to get the problem
drinkers into treatment were examined. Author biographical information. Abstract. 3 tables. 20 references.

7.068   Freedberg, Edmund J. and William E. Johnston. "Outcome
        with Alcoholics Seeking Treatment Voluntarily or after
        Confrontation by Their Employer." Journal of Occupa-
        tional Medicine 22 (1980):   83-86.

        Research done in Canada demonstrated the usefulness of
        coercion in convincing alcoholic employees to seek treat-
        ment. The Ontario Problem Assessment Battery (OPAB) was
        used by the authors. Over 400 alcoholics were studied.
        Abstract. Author biographical information. 9 tables.
        18 references.

7.069   Friedman, Lisa Adrian. "Differential Family Recovery in
        Alcoholism." Dissertation Abstracts International 41:
        4661B. Ph.D. dissertation, California School of Profes-
        sional Psychology, Berkeley, 1980. Order No. DA8110154.

        Sixteen families were studied within the framework of
        the Circumplex Model of Family Systems, a description of
        families in terms of adaptability and cohesion. The au-
        thor was interested in how the entire family changed, as
        the alcoholic member of the family made the transition
        to abstinence.

7.070   "Fructose Treatment of Acute Alcohol Intoxication." Nu-
        trition Reviews 36 (January 1978):   14-15.

        Twenty men between the ages of eighteen and seventy, ex-
        hibiting acute alcohol intoxication, participated in a
        study in which fructose was used to treat the alcohol
        intoxication. The study revealed that fructose has no
        proven benefits over glucose because of side effects as-
        sociated with the fructose treatment. Abstract. 1 ref-
        erence.

7.071   Fuller, Richard K. and Harold P. Roth. "Disulfiram for
        the Treatment of Alcoholism: An Evaluation in 128 Men."
        Annals of Internal Medicine 90 (June 1979):   901-904.

        Patients at the Cleveland, Ohio Veterans Administration
        Hospital were the subjects for this study. The subjects
        were randomly assigned to one of three treatment groups.
        Two groups were control groups. Disulfiram was found to
        be of value in treating alcoholism. Author biographical
        information. Abstract. 2 tables. 15 references.

7.072   Gallant, Donald M. "Does Lithium Have Value in the
        Treatment of Alcoholism?" Alcoholism: Clinical and Ex-
        perimental Research 9 (May-June 1985):   297-298.

        Attempts to determine the effectiveness of lithium in
        treating alcoholism. Author biographical information. 2
        references.

7.073   Gallen, Melvin. "A Follow-Up Evaluation of Two

Contrasting Alcoholic Treatment Programs." _Dissertation Abstracts International_ 35: 3578B. Ph.D. dissertation, University of Houston, 1974. Order No. DA751030.

This research involved alcoholic patients at the Veterans Administration Hospital in Houston, Texas. A behavior therapy alcoholism treatment program was compared to more traditional treatment.

7.074   Garcia, Reginaldo G. "Personality and Alcoholism Treatment." _Dissertation Abstracts International_ 46: 3592B. Ph.D. dissertation, University of Colorado at Boulder, 1985. Order No. DA8528485.

The purpose of the author's investigation was to determine if psychological treatment can be improved by having the treatment "fit" the alcoholic's personality. Four concepts--personal characteristics, behavior, significance, and performance--helped provide a conceptual understanding of personality.

7.075   Gerson, Amy Cohen. "Demographic and Drinking Variables Correlated with Visits to Aftercare for Alcoholic Males and Females." _Dissertation Abstracts International_ 46: 112B. Ph.D. dissertation, Kent State University, 1984. Order No. DA8505893.

Male and female alcoholics in Lorain, Ohio were the research sample. The men and women were patients at the Lakeland Institute. The patients were studied in relation to fifteen demographic and drinking variables. The research revealed that a higher percentage of women than men attended aftercare.

7.076   Gillham, M. Beth, Katherine Southworth and Jamie Dollahite. "Nutritional Treatment for the Alcoholic Patient." _CCQ_ 8 (March 1986): 20-28.

Nutritional status and alcohol intake, the metabolic effects of alcohol, cirrhosis, and hepatic encephalopathy are covered. Oral, enteral, or parenteral nourishment will be necessary, depending on the individual patient. Nurse and dietician will often work together to provide optimal nutritional care. Author biographical information. 39 references.

7.077   Gitlow, Stanley E. and Herbert S. Peyser. "Appendix A: Sedative-Hypnotic Drugs." in _Alcoholism: A Practical Treatment Guide_, edited by Stanley E. Gitlow and Herbert S. Peyser, 245. New York, NY: Grune and Stratton, Inc., 1980.

Lists three categories of drugs used in treating alcoholism. The first category--barbiturates, two examples of which are amytal and seconal. The second category--

benzadiazepines which are known as minor tranquilizers. Four examples of these are: librium, serax, dalmane, and tranzene. The third category includes a number of other drugs. Five examples are: miltown, somnor, doriden, noludar, and milpath.

7.078   Gitlow, Stanley E. and Herbert S. Peyser. "Appendix C: AMA Guidelines for Alcoholism: Diagnosis, Treatment and Referral." in Alcoholism: A Practical Treatment Guide, edited by Stanley E. Gitlow and Herbert S. Peyser, 267-272. New York, NY: Grune and Stratton, Inc., 1980.

These guidelines were adopted on October 8-9, 1979 by the American Medical Association Council on Scientific Affairs. Each of the guidelines include explanatory notes.

7.079   Glaser, Frederick B. and Alan C. Ogborne. "Does A.A. Really Work?" British Journal of Addiction 77 (1982): 123-129.

Five reasons for asking the question: does A.A. really work? States how this question could be answered. Author biographical information. 21 references.

7.080   Goodwin, Donald W. "Alcoholics Anonymous." Chapter in Alcoholism: The Facts, by Donald W. Goodwin, 106-115. Oxford: Oxford University Press, 1981.

Looks at the effectiveness of Alcoholics Anonymous (AA) which was created in 1935.

7.081   Goodwin, Donald W. "Attacking the Problem." Chapter in Alcoholism: The Facts, by Donald W. Goodwin, 116-129. Oxford: Oxford University Press, 1981.

Role of the family, employer, doctor, and society in combating alcoholism.

7.082   Goodwin, Donald W. "Specific Treatments." Chapter in Alcoholism: The Facts, by Donald W. Goodwin, 88-105. Oxford: Oxford University Press, 1981.

Specific treatments for alcoholism include psychotherapy, behavior therapy, and drug therapy.

7.083   Googins, Bradley Kenneth. "The Use and Implementation of Occupational Alcoholism Programs by Supervisors: An Analysis of Barriers." Dissertation Abstracts International 40: 2269A-2270A. Ph.D. dissertation, Brandeis University, 1979. Order No. DA7922701.

Eighty corporate supervisors took part in this study. Forty supervisors had referred employees to the company

alcoholism program, forty had not made any referrals.
The author was interested in differences between these
two types of supervisors. One difference was that referring supervisors were significantly older. Another
difference was that non-referring supervisors were better liked than referring supervisors.

7.084   Grant, Marcus and Bruce Ritson. "What Can Be Achieved
        through Treatment?" Chapter in Alcohol: The Prevention
        Debate, by Marcus Grant and Bruce Ritson, 25-32. Lon-
        don: Croom Helm Ltd., 1983.

        An examination of preventive strategies--primary, sec-
        ondary, and tertiary--applied to alcohol problems.

7.085   Greer, Richard M. and William M. Prado. "Stimulating
        Participation in an Alcohol Treatment Program through
        Videotape Modeling." Newsletter for Research in Mental
        Health and Behavioral Sciences 15 (November 1973): 34-
        35.

        The research setting was the North Little Rock Veterans
        Administration Hospital in North Little Rock, Arkansas.
        Videotape modeling treatment was a successful way of
        stimulating participation in the alcohol treatment pro-
        gram. Some of the indicators of success were: reduced
        neurotic symptomatology, reduced anxiety, more self-con-
        fidence, and a greater desire and motivation to remain
        sober. Author biographical information.

7.086   Groupe, Vincent. "Addresses of Rehabilitation Centers."
        in Alcoholism Rehabilitation: Methods and Experiences
        of Private Rehabilitation Centers, edited by Vincent
        Groupe, 131. New Brunswick, NJ: Rutgers Center of Alco-
        hol Studies, 1978.

        Gives the addresses of the following thirteen alcoholism
        rehabilitation centers: (1) Alcoholic Clinic of Youngs-
        town (Youngstown, Ohio), (2) Carrier Clinic (Belle Mead,
        New Jersey), (3) Chit Chat Farms (Wernersville, Pennsyl-
        vania), (4) Cumberland Heights (Nashville, Tennessee),
        (5) Gateway Rehabilitation Center (Aliquippa, Pennsyl-
        vania), (6) Hazelden Foundation (Center City, Minnesota),
        (7) Little Company of Mary Hospital (Evergreen Park, Il-
        linois), (8) Little Hill-Alina Lodge (Blairstown, New
        Jersey), (9) Livengrin Foundation (Eddington, Pennsyl-
        vania), (10) Alcoholism Treatment Center (Park Ridge, Il-
        linois), (11) Smithers Alcoholism Treatment and Train-
        ing Center (New York, New York), (12) Starlite Village
        Hospital (Center Point, Texas), and (13) Willingway Hos-
        pital (Statesboro, Georgia).

7.087   Gusfield, Joseph R. "The Prevention of Drinking Prob-
        lems." Chapter in Alcohol and Alcohol Problems: New
        Thinking and New Directions, edited by William J.

Filstead, Jean J. Rossi and Mark Keller, 267-291. Cambridge, MA: Ballinger Publishing Co., 1976.

Policies aimed at the prevention of drinking problems can target levels of consumption, persuasion, and the screening of individuals. Political, cultural, legal, and communication variables come into play. This chapter was originally a paper presented at the Lutheran General Hospital's Symposium on Alcoholism and Alcohol Problems, Park Ridge, Illinois, Spring 1973. 11 footnotes. 46 references.

7.088   Gwinner, Paul. "Treatment Approaches." Chapter in Alcoholism in Perspective, edited by Marcus Grant and Paul Gwinner, 113-121. London: Croom Helm Ltd., 1979.

Differentiates between and discusses the medical and dimensional models of alcoholism treatment.

7.089   Halikas, James A. "Psychotropic Medication Used in the Treatment of Alcoholism." Hospital and Community Psychiatry 34 (1983): 1035-1039.

Phenothiazines, benzodiazepines, monoamine oxidase inhibitors, lithium, metronidazole, pentothal, propranolol, and disulfiram. These drugs are viewed as adjuncts to social and behavioral treatment of alcoholism. Drug therapy in itself is not effective and not recommended. Author biographical information. Abstract. 57 references.

7.090   Hamburg, Sam. "Behavior Therapy in Alcoholism: A Critical Review of Broad-Spectrum Approaches." Journal of Studies on Alcohol 36 (1975): 69-87.

Broad-spectrum approaches are more effective than conventional methods in the behavior therapy of alcoholism, and, for some alcoholics, controlled drinking is a reasonable treatment goal. Author biographical information. Abstract. 67 references.

7.091   Hamilton, Margaret. "Treatment of Working Alcoholics." Occupational Health 28 (1976): 398-399.

Dr. Boris Serebro established the first outpatient clinic in Britain to treat employed alcoholics. The clinic is part of the Central Middlesex Industrial Health Service.

7.092   Hansen, James. "Sobering-Up Drug Can Cancel Alcohol as an Intoxicant." Science Digest 88 (July 1980): 55-57.

A research team headed by Dr. William Jeffcoate, an endocrinologist at Nottingham City Hospital, in England, used the drug naloxone to block the intoxicating effects

of alcohol. The other members of the team: Michael
Herbert, Andrew Hastings, Christine Walder and Michael
Cullen. Twenty doctors were the subjects for the
naloxone study.

7.093   Harrison, Kit William. "Engaging the Male Inpatient
Alcoholic in Treatment through the Reduction of Psychological Stress: An Application of Stress Inoculation
Therapy." Dissertation Abstracts International 43:
4147B. Ph.D. dissertation, University of Missouri, Columbia, 1982. Order No. DA8310396.

Stress inoculation therapy (SIT) was found to be beneficial to alcoholics taking part in a six-week, veterans administration alcoholism program. The Minnesota
Multiphasic Personality Inventory (MMPI) was used to
test fifty-four alcoholics for stress.

7.094   Harwin, Judith and Linda Hunt. "Working with Alcohol-
ics." Chapter in Alcoholism in Perspective, edited by
Marcus Grant and Paul Gwinner, 143-158. London: Croom
Helm Ltd., 1979.

A feature of this chapter is dialogue between an inter-
viewer and an alcoholic. The purpose of the dialogue
is to illustrate characteristics of the helping process.

7.095   Heather, B.B. "The Crisis in the Treatment of Alcohol
Abuse." in Aspects of Alcohol and Drug Dependence, edited by J.S. Madden, Robin Walker and W.H. Kenyon, 252-
259. Kent: Pitman Medical Ltd., 1980.

Kuhnian paradigm change, as discussed in The Structure
of Scientific Revolutions, a book by Thomas Kuhn, is
related to the treatment of alcohol abuse. This paper
is based on the Proceedings of the Fourth International
Conference on Alcoholism and Drug Dependence, Liverpool,
England. 15 references.

7.096   Hedberg, Allan G. and Lowell Campbell, III. "A Comparison of Four Behavioral Treatments of Alcoholism." Journal of Behavior Therapy and Experimental Psychiatry 5
(December 1974): 251-256.

Systematic desensitization, covert sensitization, electric shock, and behavioral family counseling were the
four behavior therapy approaches compared for therapeutic
efficacy. Forty-nine alcoholics--forty-five males and
four females--were the study sample. Behavioral family
counseling proved to be the most effective alcoholism
treatment method. Author biographical information. Abstract. 1 table. 31 references.

7.097   Heringer, Michael P. "Workers' Compensation: Should
Intoxication Bar Recovery? Montana Law Review 46

(Summer 1985):   419-432.

Examines the effect of intoxication on workers' compensation law in Montana and focuses on three intoxication
defense standards.   71 footnotes.

7.098   Hertzman, Marc.   "Getting Alcoholics Out of Your Office,
into Treatment, and Back to Your Office."   Primary Care
6 (June 1979):   403-416.

Five major topics: the etiology of alcohol-related syndromes, identifying and confronting alcoholics, office
treatment of alcoholism, detoxification as an office
procedure, and what to do to keep the alcoholic in treatment.   This information is intended primarily for the
family practitioner.   Author biographical information.
Abstract.   1 table.   20 references.

7.099   Hertzman, Marc and Barrie Montague.   "Cost-Benefit Analysis and Alcoholism."   Journal of Studies on Alcohol 38
(1977):   1371-1385.

The authors contend that cost-benefit analysis is a valuable planning tool in alcoholism treatment.   Author biographical information.   3 tables.   6 footnotes.   24 references.   Abstract.

7.100   Hodgson, Ray.   "Much Ado about Nothing Much: Alcoholism
Treatment and the Rand Report."   British Journal of Addiction 74 (1979):   227-234.

Comments on a 1976 Rand Corp. report on controlled drinking.   The report stated that controlled drinking was desirable for some alcoholics.   A considerable amount of
controversy resulted from this suggestion.   Author biographical information.   12 references.

7.101   Hodgson, Ray J.   "Behavioural Psychotherapy."   Chapter in
Alcoholism in Perspective, edited by Marcus Grant and
Paul Gwinner, 122-131.   London: Croom Helm Ltd., 1979.

The emphasis in this chapter is on reducing the proba-
bility of compulsive drinking by modifying antecedent
cues and by modifying consequences.   2 figures.

7.102   Holden, Constance.   "Rand Issues Final Alcoholism Report."   Science 207 (February 1980):   855-856.

Remarks about a report by Rand Corp. researchers.   The
report concerns alcoholism treatment, was funded by the
National Institute on Alcohol Abuse and Alcoholism
(NIAAA), and cost over half a million dollars.   The report contends that controlled drinking may be feasible
for less severe cases of alcoholism.   J. Michael Polich,
a sociologist, is the main Rand Corp. author of the

report.

7.103   Holmes, Elaine Davies. "A Comparison of Three Aversive
        Conditioning Paradigms in the Treatment of Alcoholism."
        Dissertation Abstracts International 32: 6049B. Ph.D.
        dissertation, University of Utah, 1972. Order No. DA-
        7212669.

        Male veteran alcoholics were the sample for this inves-
        tigation. The Sepulveda Veterans Administration Hospi-
        tal was the setting for the research. Five conditioning
        paradigms were used. It was concluded that a patient's
        personality should be taken into account before a con-
        ditioning paradigm is selected.

7.104   Hopson, Anna Lee. "Where Are the Other Victims of Alco-
        holism?" Labor-Management Alcoholism Journal 7 (Septem-
        ber-October 1977): 22-23.

        Employed spouses, parents, and children of alcoholics
        are also victims of alcoholism. Sick leave costs for
        these people are extremely high, yet very few of these
        people are referred for treatment. Employee alcoholism
        program directors need new approaches to deal with this
        problem. Author biographical information. 1 photo-
        graph.

7.105   "How an EAP Works." Benefits Canada 7 (July-August
        1983): 20 and 22.

        Provides information about employee assistance programs
        (EAPs) in Canada. Includes comments by Donald Henderson
        (William M. Mercer), Wayne Ogg (Addiction Research Foun-
        dation of Ontario), and Anthea Stewart (Thorne Steven-
        son and Kellogg). 1 illustration.

7.106   Hunt, Linda and Judith Harwin. "Social Work Theory and
        Practice." Chapter in Alcoholism in Perspective, edited
        by Marcus Grant and Paul Gwinner, 132-142. London:
        Croom Helm Ltd., 1979.

        Covers social work theory and practice in relation to
        helping the alcoholic. Covers, more specifically, the
        alcoholic's social situation, assessment of his needs,
        and establishment of a relationship with him. A table
        summarizes frameworks for assessing the alcoholic from
        the viewpoint of psychosocial therapy, crisis theory,
        and the systems approach to family therapy. 2 tables.

7.107   Imber, S., E. Schultz, F. Funderburk, R. Allen and R.
        Flamer. "The Fate of the Untreated Alcoholic: Toward
        a Natural History of the Disorder." Journal of Nervous
        and Mental Disease 162 (1976): 238-247.

        Reports on male alcoholics who were studied initially

and at one-year and three-year follow-ups. Overall outcome, abstinence outcome, type of resources in relation
to outcome, and mortality outcome were determined.
Eighty-three subjects were interviewed initially. Seventy-three were located for the three-year follow-up.
Author biographical information. 5 tables. 2 figures.
9 references. 3 footnotes.

7.108   "Insurance Group Lauds Alcoholism Presentation." Labor-
Management Alcoholism Newsletter 2 (March-April 1973):
14-17.

Comments on a presentation about group health insurance
coverage for alcoholism. The presentation was held at
the Annual Meeting, Health Insurance Association of America, Montreal, Quebec, April 1973.

7.109   Jabbonsky, Larry. "What Wholesalers Have to Say about
Alcohol Abuse." Beverage World 104 (December 1985):
57.

How beer wholesalers can help solve the alcohol abuse
problem. The wholesalers spoke at the 1985 National
Beer Wholesalers Association (NBWA) convention. The
wholesalers were from Michigan, Virginia, California,
Illinois, and Colorado. 5 photographs.

7.110   John, Ulrich. "Some Career Aspects of Alcoholics Not
Motivated to Take Part in Therapy 6 Months after Detoxification." Drug and Alcohol Dependence 16 (December
1985): 279-285.

Alcoholics in West Germany were the subjects. A total
of forty-seven alcoholics, divided into two groups, were
compared regarding career and lack of motivation to participate in therapy six months after detoxification.
Alcohol dependence, social decline, balance (positive
versus negative life features), and subjective perspective (of the alcoholic) were investigated. Author biographical information. Abstract. 1 table. 1 figure.
10 references.

7.111   Johnson, Vernon E. "Counseling Alcoholics." Chapter
in I'll Quit Tomorrow, by Vernon E. Johnson, Revised
Edition, 101-108. New York, NY: Harper and Row, Publishers, Inc., 1980.

Common problems encountered by people who counsel alcoholics. Problems arise not only between alcoholics and
counselors, but also between different professionals,
representing different disciplines. Psychiatrists,
clergymen, psychologists, and social workers may, particularly when working as a team, differ on counseling
techniques. 1 figure.

7.112   Kay, Richard Steven. "Alcoholism Relapse among Alcohol-
        ics Anonymous Participants." Dissertation Abstracts In-
        ternational 47: 2141B. Ph.D. dissertation, United
        States International University, 1985. Order No. DA86-
        17918.

        The Alcoholic Profile Questionnaire was administered to
        Alcoholics Anonymous (AA) participants in this study
        which tested four variables. Ethanol consumption and
        Alcoholics Anonymous attendance were the best predictors
        of relapse rates.

7.113   Kruzich, David John. "An Examination of Client and Pro-
        gram Related Variables as Predictors of Alcohol Treat-
        ment Outcomes." Dissertation Abstracts International
        41: 2296A. Ph.D. dissertation, University of Minneso-
        ta, 1980. Order No. DA8025472.

        Individuals admitted to Meadowbrook Treatment Center, a
        Hennepin County Program, were the client sample for this
        investigation. Alcoholics Anonymous (AA) affiliation,
        employment, family functioning, and other variables were
        assessed at three follow-up intervals. Stepwise Multi-
        ple Regression was used to analyze data.

7.114   Kurtz, Ernest. Not-God: A History of Alcoholics Anony-
        mous. Center City, MN: Hazelden Educational Services,
        1979.

        This book is based on archival research, alcoholism lit-
        erature, interviews, and attendance at Alcoholics Anony-
        mous (AA) meetings. Nine chapters cover the history of
        AA, beginning with its establishment in 1934.

7.115   Kurtz, Norman R., Bradley Googins and Carol Williams.
        "Clients' Views of an Alcoholism Program." Labor-Manage-
        ment Alcoholism Journal 10 (November-December 1980): 102
        and 107-113.

        Compares the views of individuals who participated in an
        occupational alcoholism program (OAP) with the views of
        OAP personnel. Thirty-nine employees of a public utility
        in the U.S. northeast took part in a OAP. There were
        twenty-nine males and ten females. Four areas for fur-
        ther research are indicated. 1 table. 2 footnotes. 20
        references.

7.116   Lanyon, Richard I., Richard V. Primo, Francis Terrell and
        Albert Wener. "An Aversion-Desensitization Treatment
        for Alcoholism." Journal of Consulting and Clinical
        Psychology 38, No. 3 (1972): 394-398.

        Male alcoholic patients, at the Mayview State Hospital in
        Pennsylvania, volunteered to take part in this research.
        Each volunteer was treated with one of three types of

treatment: aversion therapy, systematic desensitization,
or contact control. Research tools included: the Minnesota Multiphasic Personality Inventory (MMPI), MacAndrew Alcoholism Scale, the Fear Survey Schedule IV, and
the Alcadd Test. Author biographical information. Abstract. 3 tables. 14 references.

7.117   Lawson, Gary, James S. Peterson and Ann Lawson. "Treatment Approaches to Alcoholism." Chapter in Alcoholism
and the Family: A Guide to Treatment and Prevention, by
Gary Lawson, James S. Peterson and Ann Lawson, 17-29.
Rockville, MD: Aspen Systems Corp., 1983.

Reviews three alcoholism treatment models: Alcoholics
Anonymous (AA), transactional analysis, and behavioral.
1 table. 8 references.

7.118   Layne, Norman R. and George D. Lowe. "The Impact of
Loss of Career Continuity on the Later Occupational Ad-
justment of Problem Drinkers." Journal of Health and
Social Behavior 20 (June 1979): 187-193.

This is the revision of a paper presented at the Annual
Meeting, American Sociological Association, New York,
August 29-September 3, 1976. Nearly 500, white, male
alcoholics were the sample. These subjects were categorized into four occupational status categories: upper
white collar, lower white collar, upper blue collar,
lower blue collar. All these alcoholics were admitted
to a voluntary treatment clinic. Author biographical
information. Abstract. 2 tables. 2 notes. 26 references.

7.119   Levy, Marguerite F., Walter Reichman and Stephen Herrington. "Abstinent Alcoholics' Adjustment to Work." Journal of Studies on Alcohol 42 (1981): 529-532.

Abstinent alcoholics were studied 3.5 and 6.5 years after treatment. These alcoholics were better adjusted
to work 6.5 years after treatment than 3.5 years after
having been treated. Author biographical information.
Abstract. 11 references.

7.120   Levy, Richard, Tom Elo and Irwin B. Hanenson. "Intrave-
nous Fructose Treatment of Acute Alcohol Intoxication."
Archives of Internal Medicine 137 (September 1977):
1175-1177.

This study took place at the Cincinnati, Ohio General
Hospital. It was a double-blind study and involved twenty male subjects. The subjects were treated with glu-
cose and fructose. The researchers concluded that fructose not be used for treating acute alcohol intoxication.
Author biographical information. Abstract. 2 figures.
1 table. 19 references.

7.121   Lewis, Marvin W. "An Analysis of the Self Concept Scores
        of Low Income Black Alcoholics in Dissonant and Consonant
        Treatment Settings." Dissertation Abstracts Internation-
        al 46: 1324B. Ph.D. dissertation, Brandeis University,
        1985. Order No. DA8509080.

        Male and female alcoholics in Westchester County, New
        York participated in this study. The thirty-five sub-
        jects were tested by means of the Tennessee Self Concept
        Scale, Michigan Alcoholism Screening Test (MAST), and
        the Definitions of Alcoholism Scale. An important re-
        search finding was that there should be separate treat-
        ment programs for the two sexes. Different treatment
        needs exist for men and women.

7.122   Lindsay, Wanda P. "The Role of the Occupational Thera-
        pist Treatment of Alcoholism." American Journal of Oc-
        cupational Therapy 37 (January 1983): 36-43.

        After a look at the incidence of alcoholism, this arti-
        cle talks about the physiological and psychosocial ef-
        fects of alcohol, then discusses alcoholism as a dis-
        ease. This is followed by a description of the Alcohol-
        ism Treatment Unit at the Mercy Hospital and Medical
        Center in Chicago. The work of the occupational thera-
        pist in this context is highlighted. Craft activities
        and recreation are two types of therapy used. Author
        biographical information. Abstract. 2 figures. 36
        references.

7.123   Loweree, Frank, Steven Freng and Beatrice C. Barnes.
        "Admitting an Intoxicated Patient." American Journal
        of Nursing 84 (1984): 616-618.

        Elaborates on strategies nurses can use to effectively
        admit intoxicated patients to the hospital. Quick think-
        ing by hospital staff is a major requisite when dealing
        with these patients. Author biographical information.
        1 illustration.

7.124   Luks, Allan. "Alcoholism: Do Threats and Therapy Mix?"
        Hastings Center Report 12 (December 1982): 7-11.

        Individual rights and society's efforts to control alco-
        holism in the U.S., Czechoslovakia, Poland, Finland,
        Canada, Yugoslavia, and other countries. Author bio-
        graphical information.

7.125   Lundquist, Gunnar A.R. "Strategies and Goals in the
        Treatment and Control of Alcoholism." in Alcoholism:
        A Medical Profile, Proceedings of the First Internation-
        al Medical Conference on Alcoholism, London, September
        10-14, 1973, 168-172. London: B. Edsall and Co. Ltd.,
        1974.

Five main types of alcoholic individuals and the appro-
priate treatment for each type. French abstract. German abstract.

7.126   MacDonald, John J. "The Key Role of the Alcoholism
Volunteer." Labor-Management Alcoholism Journal 10
(May-June 1981): 228-229.

Supports volunteer work in fighting alcoholism. Author
biographical information.

7.127   MacDonell, Frank J. "Alcoholism in the Workplace: Differential Diagnosis." Occupational Health Nursing 29
(March 1981): 14-16.

Physical symptoms, signs and symptoms of withdrawal, behavioral symptoms, and differential treatment. Author
biographical information. 1 photograph.

7.128   Machado, Gerardo Antonio. "A Multimodal Burnout Prevention and Reduction Program for Alcoholism Counselors." Dissertation Abstracts International 43: 4154B.
PSY.D. dissertation, Rutgers University the State University of New Jersey, 1982. Order No. DA8310994.

Thirteen alcoholism program staff members took part in
a six-week program for the prevention of burnout. The
participants completed the Maslach Burnout Inventory before and after the pilot program. A Session Satisfaction Questionnaire was also used.

7.129   Marks, Vida L. "Health Teaching for Recovering Alcoholic Patients." American Journal of Nursing 80 (1980):
2058-2061.

Describes an alcoholism treatment program at the Brent-
wood Veterans Administration Hospital, Los Angeles. The
program includes both inpatient treatment and an outpatient program. The article covers: the early days of
sobriety, the second week of sobriety, and the third to
fifth week of sobriety. Teaching principles and a se-
lection of topics regarding the recovering alcoholic patient are also included. Author biographical information. 3 sketches. 9 references.

7.130   Marotta-Sims, Janetti. "The Effect of Marital Status,
Marriage Characteristics, and Demographic Variables on
Alcohol Inpatient Treatment Completion." Dissertation
Abstracts International 46: 4407B. Ph.D. dissertation,
Univeristy of Nevada, Reno, 1985. Order No. DA8601812.

Over a thousand alcoholic, male, veterans administration
inpatients were the sample for this research. The purpose of the author's investigation was to examine marital
status and marriage characteristics as they relate to

treatment completion for alcoholics. There were two parts to this study. One thousand and seventy subjects participated in the first part. Seventy-three subjects participated in the second part.

7.131   Mastrich, James L., Jr. "Influences on the Successful Treatment of Alcoholics Referred through Employee Assistance Programs." Dissertation Abstracts International 46: 3251B. ED.D. dissertation, Rutgers University the State University of New Jersey, New Brunswick, 1985. Order No. DA8524231.

Employee assistance program (EAP) staff from ten organizations were interviewed to obtain data for this research. Information on over 300 subjects was gathered. The author was very interested in finding out what prompted employees to participate in EAPs.

7.132   Maxwell, Milton A. "Alcoholics Anonymous." Chapter in Alcohol, Science and Society Revisited, edited by Edith Lisansky Gomberg, Helene Raskin White and John A. Carpenter, 295-305. Ann Arbor, MI: University of Michigan Press, 1982.

Gives a short account of Alcoholics Anonymous (AA) in the early 1940s then focuses on this organization in the early 1980s, describing its growth over forty years. 7 references.

7.133   Maxwell, Milton A. The Alcoholics Anonymous Experience: A Close-Up View for Professionals. New York, NY: McGraw-Hill Book Co., 1984.

First person experiences illustrate what happens at Alcoholics Anonymous (AA) meetings, what members find in the AA fellowship, how they feel about it, and how the experience affects their recovery and lives. The author researched Alcoholics Anonymous members throughout the U.S. and Canada.

7.134   Mayer, William. "Alcohol Abuse and Alcoholism: The Psychologist's Role in Prevention, Research, and Treatment." American Psychologist 38 (October 1983): 1116-1121.

Areas covered: defining and diagnosing alcoholism, treatment, identification of persons at high risk for alcohol problems, the workplace, the military, children of alcoholic parents, and adolescents. Author biographical information. 1 photograph.

7.135   McAfee, Raymond Mack. "Male and Female Abstainers Attending Alcoholics Anonymous: Their Adjustments in Personality Structure, Cognitive Orientation, and Interpersonal Relationships." Dissertation Abstracts

International 41: 2020A. ED.D. dissertation, University of Houston, 1980. Order No. DA8027013.

One hundred and ten men and women, who abstained from alcohol, volunteered to take part in this investigation. Each participant was administered the Sixteen Personality Factor Questionnaire (16PF), Form A; Dogmatism Scale (DS), Form E; and Interpersonal Check List (ICL). This study revealed that both types of abstainers, male and female, exhibited evidence of pathology in their post-drinking personality.

7.136   McCarthy, John Michael. "The Prevalence of Hopelessness in Hospitalized Alcoholics." *Dissertation Abstracts International* 41: 4676B. ED.D. dissertation, Western Michigan University, 1981. Order No. DA8112340.

This research was the first study of hopelessness in alcoholics. The subjects were ninety-four inpatients at the Veterans Administration Medical Center in Battle Creek, Michigan. Each subject completed the Hopelessness Scale (HS), Beck Depression Inventory (BDI), and the Michigan Alcoholism Screening Test (MAST). The researcher was interested in hopelessness and a variety of variables, including severity of alcoholism, age, number of hospitalizations for drinking, and pending legal problems.

7.137   McLatchie, Brian H., Pauline M. Grey and Yvonne S. Johns. "A Model for Alcohol Clinics Working with Industry." *Canada's Mental Health* 29 (March 1981): 20-22 and 33.

Pinewood Centre (Oshawa General Hospital) in Oshawa, Ontario is an alcoholism treatment facility which became involved with industry to treat occupational alcoholism. Author biographical information. 1 figure. 8 references.

7.138   Meyer, Malcolm. "The Systems Approach to Alcoholism." *Labor-Management Alcoholism Journal* 7 (July-August 1977): 22-23.

Endorses the systems approach to alcoholism. This approach is associated with Joseph L. Kellerman. The author states why it should be used in employee alcoholism programs (EAPs). A key feature of the systems approach is that it does not focus on determining why something happened, but on what, when, and where it happened. Author biographical information. 1 photograph.

7.139   Michaels, Andrew W. "The Prevalence of Loneliness in Alcoholic Versus Non-Alcoholic Treatment Populations." *Dissertation Abstracts International* 42: 4935B. Ph.D. dissertation, Pacific Graduate School of Psychology,

1982.   Order No. DA8212660.

The author's research led him to conclude that alcoholics seeking treatment--at a community, mental health
outpatient clinic--were not more lonely than were nonalcoholics seeking treatment for other reasons. A total sample of sixty subjects, representing both types
of individuals, participated in the research. The Bradley Loneliness Scale and the Psychological Screening Inventory were administered to the subjects.

7.140   Miller, Peter M., Michel Hersen, Richard M. Eisler and
Diana P. Hemphill. "Electrical Aversion Therapy with
Alcoholics: An Analogue Study." Behaviour Research
and Therapy 11 (1973): 491-497.

Male subjects being treated for alcoholism voluntarily,
at the Veterans Administration Center in Jackson, Mississippi, took part in this study. Ten subjects received electrical aversion conditioning; ten received
control conditioning; and ten received group therapy.
Conditioning was not the reason for the success of
electrical aversion therapy with these subjects. Author biographical information. Abstract. 3 tables.
15 references.

7.141   Miller, Sheldon I. "How to Tell if Alcoholism Treatment
Has Worked: Assessing Outcome Studies." Hospital and
Community Psychiatry 37 (June 1986): 555-556.

If an objective diagnosis of alcoholism is not made,
and the data collected is not analyzed objectively, then
it is difficult to determine the effectiveness of alcoholism treatment. Theoretical prejudices of clinicians
may influence accuracy of diagnosis. Mean corpuscular
volume (MCV), serum alcohol levels, and gamma glutamyl
transpeptidase (GGT) are among the objective physical
measurements which should be taken. Author biographical
information. 6 references.

7.142   Miller, William R. "When Is a Book a Treatment?: Bibliotherapy for Problem Drinkers." Chapter in Clinical
Case Studies in the Behavioral Treatment of Alcoholism,
edited by William M. Hay and Peter E. Nathan, 49-72.
New York, NY: Plenum Press, 1982.

Two case histories are used to illustrate bibliotherapy
in the treatment of alcoholism. 4 figures. 58 references.

7.143   Miller, William R. and Reid K. Hester. "Treating the
Problem Drinker: Modern Approaches." Chapter in The
Addictive Behaviors: Treatment of Alcoholism, Drug
Abuse, Smoking and Obesity, edited by William R. Miller,
11-141. Oxford: Pergamon Press Ltd., 1980.

Drugs, aversion therapies, hypnosis, psychotherapy, group
therapies, halfway houses, family therapy, and relaxation training are forms of alcoholism treatment covered
in this chapter. 3 tables. 1 figure. 609 references.

7.144   Miller, William R. and Cheryl A. Taylor. "Relative Ef-
fectiveness of Bibliotherapy, Individual and Group Self-
Control Training in the Treatment of Problem Drinkers."
Addictive Behaviors 5 (1980): 13-24.

Forty-one people from the Albuquerque, New Mexico area
took part in this research. Effectiveness of four forms
of behavioral self-control training (BSCT) was evaluated.
The BSCT was used to reduce alcohol consumption. Author
biographical information. Abstract. 4 figures. 4 tables. 31 references.

7.145   Miller, William R., Terry F. Pechacek and Sam Hamburg.
"Group Behavior Therapy for Problem Drinkers." International Journal of the Addictions 16 (1981): 829-839.

Twenty-eight problem drinkers from the San Jose and Palo
Alto, California area took part in behavioral self-control training (BSCT) in order to achieve moderate drinking. Therapists from the Palo Alto Veterans Administration Hospital conducted ten sessions over a period of
ten weeks. At the end of the training period, and at
follow-up, 70% of the problem drinkers had been treated
successfully. That is, they had significantly reduced
alcohol consumption. Author biographical information.
Abstract. 2 tables. 2 figures. 22 references.

7.146   Milton, Robert Peter. "Treated Alcoholics' Attitudes
toward Drinking and Their Intention to Drink Upon the
Completion of Treatment." Dissertation Abstracts International 42: 3760A. Ph.D. dissertation, University of
Pittsburgh, 1980. Order No. DA8202333.

Two studies, involving 396 alcoholic subjects, helped
validate the Fishbein and Ajzen model for predicting
behavior.

7.147   Monk, Joshua J. "Alcoholism--The Salvation Army's Role
as a Branch of the Church." in Fifth Annual Alberta
Alcohol and Drug Research Symposium, edited by R.W.
Nutter and B.K. Sinha, 66-81. Edmonton: Alberta Alcoholism and Drug Abuse Commission, 1973.

Role of the Salvation Army in Canada in helping rehabilitate alcoholics. A four-fold program involves physical, social, mental, and spiritual elements. The Salvation Army helps alcoholics, who demonstrate progress
in rehabilitation, find work. Abstract. 1 footnote.
1 reference.

7.148   Munter, Pamela Nancy Osborne. "The Prediction of Sobri-
        ety in Alcoholics Using Four Measures of Empathy." Dis-
        sertation Abstracts International 33: 1801B. Ph.D.
        dissertation, University of Nebraska, 1972. Order No.
        DA7227415.

        Male alcoholics at the Veterans Administration Hospital
        in Lincoln, Nebraska were the subjects for this study of
        empathy and sobriety regarding alcoholics.

7.149   Nathan, Peter E. "Aversion Therapy in the Treatment of
        Alcoholism: Success and Failure." Annals of the New
        York Academy of Sciences 443 (1985): 357-364.

        A behavioral approach to treat alcoholism was first used
        in 1929. Electric shock and nausea-inducing drugs have
        been used to induce aversion to alcohol. Further re-
        search is required to determine the overall usefulness
        of lithium carbonate as an aversive agent in treating
        alcoholism. Author biographical information. Abstract.
        35 references.

7.150   "New Alcoholism Program Aims at Early Diagnosis." Busi-
        ness Insurance 10 (December 13, 1976): 60.

        American International Group, Inc. and USLIFE Corp. pro-
        vided a grant to establish Personal Consultation Ser-
        vices, an alcoholism treatment program. The program is
        available at the Beekman Downtown Hospital in Manhattan
        and the program's director is John J. Dolan.

7.151   "New Film Is Education Aid." Labor-Management Alcohol-
        ism Journal 4 (January-February 1975): 41.

        "The First Step" is a film about alcoholism and can be
        used for employee education and information. This film
        was made by Richard S. Milbauer Productions of New York.
        1 photograph.

7.152   Nussbaum, Kurt, Alan R. Kacsur, Abraham Schneidmuhl and
        John W. Shaffer. "'Hidden' Alcoholism among Disability
        Insurance Applicants: Prevalence and Degree of Impair-
        ment." Military Medicine 141 (September 1976): 596-
        599.

        Goes into detail why it is extremely difficult to find
        reference to alcoholism in many medical case records.
        Medical conditions typically associated with alcoholism
        will be indicated--alcoholism will not. Schizophrenia,
        organic brain syndrome, cirrhosis of the liver, and
        chronic pancreatitis often coexist with alcoholism. Au-
        thor biographical information. 2 tables. 6 references.

7.153   O'Connor, Art and Joan Daly. "Alcoholics: A Twenty
        Year Follow-Up Study." British Journal of Psychiatry

146 (1985):   645-647.

The authors were interested in contacting, twenty years later, individuals who had been patients treated for alcoholism at the St. John of God Hospital in Dublin, Ireland. Letters, telephone calls, police assistance, house calls, and death certificate registration information were methods used to contact former patients. The authors were most interested in drinking pattern outcome, morbidity, and mortality. Fifty-three of the 133 alcoholics treated in 1964 had died during the follow-up period. Abstract. Author biographical information. 1 appendix. 10 references.

7.154   Palangio, Jennifer Susan. "Attitudes of Psychologists toward Alcoholics." Dissertation Abstracts International 46: 3228B. Ph.D. dissertation, California School of Professional Psychology, Berkeley, 1985. Order No. DA-8522986.

Two hundred and fifty psychologists, representing the areas of teaching, research, clinical practice and administration, took part in this research. They completed two questionnaires: the Attitudes toward Alcoholics Questionnaire and the Background Questionnaire. One of the research findings was that psychologists reject the alcoholic stereotype. Another research finding was that psychologists do not believe in a poor prognosis for alcoholics.

7.155   Palkon, Dennis S. "Conjoint Alcohol Family Therapy Services for Occupational Alcoholism Programs." Labor-Management Alcoholism Journal 9 (September-October 1979): 55-62 and 65-67.

Analyzes alcoholism treatment approaches, reviews literature on conjoint alcohol family therapy, examines the role of labor and management regarding conjoint services, offers information on how to implement conjoint alcohol family therapy services, and discusses the limitations and benefits of conjoint approaches in alcoholism. Author biographical information. 1 photograph. 29 references.

7.156   Palkon, Dennis Stanley. "An Exploratory Ecological Evaluation of an Alcoholism Treatment Program: A Methodological and Substantive Investigation." Dissertation Abstracts International 38: 5717A. Ph.D. dissertation, University of Pittsburgh, 1977. Order No. DA-7801892.

Fourteen ecological dimensions--for example, spontaneity, practical orientation, and anger and aggression-- were assessed regarding male and female alcoholics. The subjects participated in a twenty-eight day alcoholism tratment program.

7.157   Patterson, Donald G. "Alcoholism Evaluation Overview."
        in Program Evaluation: Alcohol, Drug Abuse, and Mental
        Health Services, edited by Jack Zusman and Cecil R.
        Wurster, 191-200. Lexington, MA: D.C. Heath and Co.,
        1975.

        Describes the National Institute on Alcohol Abuse and
        Alcoholism (NIAAA) alcoholism treatment, program moni-
        toring system. 2 tables. 2 notes.

7.158   Pattison, E. Mansell. "Ten Years of Change in Alcohol-
        ism Treatment and Delivery Systems." American Journal
        of Psychiatry 134 (March 1977): 261-266.

        Changes in personnel, treatment goals, populations,
        treatment methods, and delivery systems during a ten-
        year period. This paper was presented at the 129th.
        Annual Meeting, American Psychiatric Association, Miami
        Beach, Florida, May 10-14, 1976. Author biographical
        information. Abstract. 93 references.

7.159   Peachey, John E. "A Review of the Clinical Use of
        Disulfiram and Calcium Carbimide in Alcoholism Treat-
        ment." Journal of Clinical Psychopharmacology 1 (No-
        vember 1981): 368-375.

        Five main topics about disulfiram and calcium carbimide
        in alcoholism treatment are discussed: their clinical
        uses, their efficacy, factors influencing treatment
        outcome, toxicity and a recommended treatment plan. Au-
        thor biographical information. Abstract. 4 tables. 1
        figure. 78 references.

7.160   Pell, Sidney and C.A. D'Alonzo. "A Five-Year Mortality
        Study of Alcoholics." Journal of Occupational Medicine
        15 (1973): 120-125.

        Premature death of alcoholics employed by E.I. du Pont
        de Nemours and Co. in Wilmington, Delaware. Mortality
        was examined in terms of drinking status, sex, socio-
        economic status, and age. The mortality of alcoholics
        was compared to the mortality of a control group. The
        mortality rate of the former group was two to three
        times higher than that of the latter group. Author
        biographical information. Abstract. 6 tables. 3 fig-
        ures. 18 references.

7.161   Peyser, Herbert S. "The Roles of the Psychiatrist, Psy-
        chologist, Social Worker, and Alcoholism Counselor."
        Chapter in Alcoholism: A Practical Treatment Guide, ed-
        ited by Stanley E. Gitlow and Herbert S. Peyser, 229-
        244. New York, NY: Grune and Stratton, Inc., 1980.

A look at the roles of the psychiatrist, psychologist, social worker, and alcoholism counselor in the treatment of alcoholism. Examines problems these professionals encounter in treating alcoholics. Includes patient case histories. 8 references.

7.162   Phillips, Haven H. "Families of Alcoholics Deserve Help, Too." Labor-Management Alcoholism Journal 9 (November-December 1979): 102-103.

Data from the St. Louis Post Office, and the Kemper Insurance Co. indicates that many people who are employed, but are not alcoholics, require counseling because they are married to or live with an alcoholic. Al-Anon Family Groups provide help to these people. The Al-Anon assistance is effective and inexpensive. Author biographical information. 2 references.

7.163   Poley, Wayne, Gary Lea and Gail Vibe. "Specific Treatment Interventions." Chapter in Alcoholism: A Treatment Manual, by Wayne Poley, Gary Lea and Gail Vibe, 61-84. New York, NY: Gardner Press, Inc., 1979.

Twenty-two specific treatment interventions for dealing with alcoholism: (1) antabuse (disulfiram), (2) minor tranquilizers and antidepressants, (3) hallucinogens, (4) biofeedback, (5) group therapy, (6) client-centered (Rogerian) therapy, (7) rational-emotive therapy (8) reality therapy, (9) transactional analysis, (10) behavior therapy, (11) aversion therapy, (12) covert sensitization, (13) hypnosis, (14) progressive relaxation training, (15) meditation, (16) systematic desensitization, (17) cognitive modification, (18) thought stopping, (19) positive self-concept enhancement, (20) assertive training, (21) social skills training, and (22) contingency contracting.

7.164   Pomerleau, Ovide F. and Ronald M. Kadden. "Behavioral Treatment Strategies for Employed Alcohol Abusers: Techniques for Moderation and Abstinence." Chapter in Occupational Clinical Psychology, edited by James S.J. Manuso, 55-68. New York, NY: Praeger Publishers, 1983.

Most relapse to uncontrolled drinking relates to negative emotional states, interpersonal conflicts, and social pressure to resume drinking. 49 references.

7.165   Powell, Barbara J., Elizabeth C. Penick, Barry I. Liskow, Audrey S. Rice and William McKnelly. "Lithium Compliance in Alcoholic Males: A Six Month Followup Study." Addictive Behaviors 11 (1986): 135-140.

Researchers at the Veterans Administration Medical Center in Kansas City, Missouri, and at the Kansas University Medical Center in Kansas City, Kansas, studied one

hundred male alcoholics. Half the patients were administered lithium carbonate; the other half were given
chlordiazepoxide. The results of using these two types
of treatment were analyzed six months later. According
to this study, lithium was not found to be an effective
means of reducing alcohol consumption. Author biographical information. Abstract. 1 figure. 1 table. 19
references.

7.166   Presnall, Lewis F. "A Neglected Means of Training on
         Alcoholism." Labor-Management Alcoholism Newsletter 2
         (September-October 1972):   20-21.

         Exposure to Alcoholics Anonymous (AA) groups is recom-
         mended to anyone who wants to work with alcoholics and
         is not a recovered alcoholic. Formal education in it-
         self is not sufficient preparation. Author biographi-
         cal information. 1 photograph.

7.167   Pritchard, Robert. "Treating the Alcoholic." Drug
         Merchandising 63 (March 1982):   30-32 and 34.

         A pharmacist discusses the medical complications of al-
         cohol abuse--cardiovascular, gastrointestinal, respira-
         tory and neurological--then talks about pharmacological
         treatment. He also comments on the fetal alcohol syn-
         drome and drug interactions with alcohol. 1 photo-
         graph. Author biographical information. 2 graphs. 3
         tables.

7.168   "Programs That Will Help You Stay on the Wagon." Busi-
         ness Week (October 26, 1981):   193-194.

         How two organizations--the Chit Chat Foundation in
         Wernersville, Pennsylvania and Alcoholics Anonymous
         (AA)--treat alcoholism.

7.169   Quinn, John C. and Gerard M. Rooney. "How to Train and
         Evaluate Employee Alcoholism Program Coordinators." La-
         bor-Management Alcoholism Journal 7 (July-August 1977):
         12-21 and 24-26.

         Detailed information about setting up the Mid-Hudson
         Region Department of Mental Hygiene Employee Alcoholism
         Program for the State of New York. Author biographical
         information. 2 photographs. 1 illustration. 2 fig-
         ures. 3 footnotes. 25 references.

7.170   Rathod, N.H. "Perception of Alcoholism." in Aspects
         of Alcohol and Drug Dependence, edited by J.S. Madden,
         Robin Walker and W.H. Kenyon, 71-76. Kent: Pitman
         Medical Ltd., 1980.

         How people in the helping professions view alcoholics.
         The attitudes of therapists have a direct bearing on

the outcome of therapy. This paper is based on the Proceedings of the Fourth International Conference on Alcoholism and Drug Dependence, Liverpool, England. 2 tables. 7 references.

7.171   Reddy, Betty. "The Family with Alcoholism in Occupational Programs." Labor-Management Alcoholism Journal
11 (July-August 1981): 36-41.

Alcoholics and family members experience similar symptoms and job behavior changes. There is a parallel
treatment plan for each. The Kemper Insurance Co. is
one company which has assisted alcoholic employees and
family members. Kemper statistics are included in this
article. 1 photograph. Author biographical information. 6 references.

7.172   Reichman, Walter, Marguerite Levy and Stephen Herrington. "Vocational Counseling in Early Sobriety." Labor-Management Alcoholism Journal 8 (March-April 1979):
192-197.

According to the authors, there are four types of alcoholics seeking vocational counseling: post-sobriety
goal setters, inappropriate career goals, uninterrupted
career pattern, and dead-end flounderers. Author biographcial information.

7.173   Rest, K.M., S. Levey, and J.R. Hall. "Instructional
Guide to Alcohol and the Workplace." Government Reports
Announcements and Index 85 (March 15, 1985): 37. NTIS
HRP-0906096/3/GAR.

Describes a videotape recommended for health professionals who deal with alcoholics and the workplace. Author biographcial information. Abstract. 2 tables.
12 references.

7.174   Ritson, E.B. "Detoxication--An Evaluation." British
Journal of Addiction Supplement No. 1, 70 (April 1975):
65-73.

Four individuals discuss detoxication. Author biographical information. 3 tables. 3 figures. 2 references.

7.175   Rivers, P. Clayton, B.P.V. Sarata and Thomas Book. "Effect of an Alcoholism Workshop on Attitudes, Job Satisfaction and Job Performance of Secretaries." Quarterly
Journal of Studies on Alcohol 35 (1974): 1382-1388.

Twenty-four secretaries in Lincoln, Nebraska participated in a workshop which improved the secretaries' job
satisfaction, job performance, and attitudes toward
clients being treated for alcoholism. The Comprehensive
Alcohol Planning Committee (CAPC) sponsored the workshop

The workshop was held during a two-day period, four
hours per day. Author biographical information. Abstract. 1 table. 6 references.

7.176   Robichaud, Colleen, Daniel Strickler, George Bigelow
        and Ira Liebson. "Disulfiram Maintenance Employee Al-
        coholism Treatment: A Three-Phase Evaluation." Be-
        haviour Research and Therapy 17 (1979): 618-621.

        Male industrial employees, who had drinking-related
        problems on the job, were treated with disulfiram.
        This treatment proved to be effective in reducing em-
        ployee absenteeism. The researchers compared absentee-
        ism rates prior to treatment, during treatment, and af-
        ter treatment. The lowest absenteeism rate was during
        treatment, the next lowest after treatment, and the
        highest prior to treatment. Abstract. Author biograph-
        ical information. 1 figure. 9 references.

7.177   Robinson, David. Talking Out of Alcoholism: The Self-
        Help Process of Alcoholics Anonymous. Baltimore, MD:
        University Park Press, 1979.

        This book is about the history, growth, and organization
        of Alcoholics Anonymous (AA), about becoming a member,
        sharing the problem of alcoholism, coping with the stig-
        ma of being an alcoholic, and Alcoholics Anonymous as a
        way of life. The book includes a survey of Alcoholics
        Anonymous in England and Wales.

7.178   Roman, Paul M. "The Emphasis on Alcoholism in Employee
        Assistance Programming: New Perspectives in an Unfin-
        ished Debate." Labor-Management Alcoholism Journal 8
        (March-April 1979): 186-191.

        The author is concerned about the decreasing emphasis
        on detecting and treating alcoholism among employees by
        means of work-based employee assistance programs (EAPs).
        Author biographical information.

7.179   Roman, Paul M. "Evaluation of Employee Alcoholism Pro-
        grams." Labor-Management Alcoholism Journal 11 (July-
        August 1981): 1-12.

        This article about the evaluation of employee alcoholism
        programs (EAPs) concentrates on two major aspects: the
        context of evaluation, and consideration of techniques
        and approaches necessary to effectively utilize evalua-
        tion concepts. Author biographical information.

7.180   Romney, D.M. and J. Bynner. "Hospital Staff's Percep-
        tions of the Alcoholic." International Journal of the
        Addictions 20 (1985): 393-402.

        Staff at the Calgary General Hospital in Calgary,

Alberta were surveyed via questionnaire to determine staff attitudes regarding four types of patients: the alcoholic, the nondrinker, the drug addict, and the heavy drinker. Types of patients were perceived in terms of: stability, dangerousness, and self-assertiveness. Author biographical information. Abstract. 4 tables. 3 figures. 8 references.

7.181   Rosenbaum, P.D. and S. Ogurzsoff. "Rationale for a Detoxication Centre." Dimensions in Health Service 54 (November 1977): 34-35.

A survey concerning the rationale for a detoxication center in Kingston, Ontario. 1 photograph. Author biographical information. 3 tables.

7.182   Rossi, Jean J. "The Agency Variable." in Treatment, by Jean J. Rossi, 23-35. Ottawa: National Planning Committee on Training of the Federal Provincial Working Group on Alcohol Problems, 1978.

Gives a systems view of agencies and people then discusses levels of intervention. This is followed by social action programs--agencies and their tasks. Some of the agencies examined: the alcoholism outpatient clinic, the alcoholism halfway house, aversion conditioning hospital, short term inpatient treatment center, the general hospital, and the mental hospital. This publication is part of a series of publications on alcohol problems in Canada. 1 figure.

7.183   Rossi, Jean J. "Methods of Intervention." in Treatment, by Jean J. Rossi, 36-61. Ottawa: National Planning Committee on Training of the Federal Provincial Working Group on Alcohol Problems, 1978.

Behavior modification, family therapy, small group methods, the therapeutic community, and Alcoholics Anonymous (AA) are the methods of intervention elaborated on. This publication is part of a series of publications on alcohol problems in Canada. 1 footnote.

7.184   Royce, James E. "Al-Anon and Alateen." Chapter in Alcohol Problems and Alcoholism: A Comprehensive Survey, by James E. Royce, 256-266. New York, NY: Free Press, 1981.

Al-Anon and Alateen are offshoots of Alcoholics Anonymous (AA). Al-Anon is for the family and friends of the alcoholic. Alateen is for children of alcoholic parents. Al-Anon was established in 1954, Alateen in 1957. 43 references.

7.185   Royce, James E. "Alcoholics Anonymous." Chapter in Alcohol Problems and Alcoholism: A Comprehensive Survey,

by James E. Royce, 242-255. New York, NY: Free Press,
1981.

How and why Alcoholics Anonymous (AA) works, even though
it is not a perfect way of treating alcoholism. Some
criticism of AA may be due to professional jealousy.
Other criticism may be due to AA's nonscientific treatment approach. This chapter includes a short history
of Alcoholics Anonymous. 38 references.

7.186   Royce, James E. "Overview of Treatments." Chapter in
Alcohol Problems and Alcoholism: A Comprehensive Sur-
vey, by James E. Royce, 225-241. New York, NY: Free
Press, 1981.

Examines numerous forms of alcoholism treatment, including detoxification, Alcoholics Anonymous (AA), antabuse
(disulfiram), aversion conditioning, chemotherapy, diet,
recreation and exercise, psychotherapy, and hypnosis.
Suggests that different forms of treatment should be
used in conjunction with one another. Claims that there
is no single, one-and-only method for treating alcoholism. 39 references.

7.187   Salum, Inna. "Treatment of Delirium Tremens." British
Journal of Addiction Supplement No. 1, 70 (April 1975):
75-80.

Six people discuss treatment of delirium tremens. Author biographical information. 2 references.

7.188   Sandin, Don. "Alcoholism: A Family Disease." Labor-
Management Alcoholism Newsletter 2 (March-April 1973):
20-22.

Al-Anon Family Groups provide assistance to families of
alcoholics. Author biographical information. 1 photograph.

7.189   Schramm, Carl J. "The Development of a Successful Alcoholism Treatment Facility." Chapter in Alcoholism and
Its Treatment in Industry, edited by Carl J. Schramm,
138-155. Baltimore, MD: Johns Hopkins University Press,
1977.

The Employee Health Program (EHP) is a treatment facility for working problem drinkers in the Baltimore area.
A number of employers and unions refer alcoholics to
this facility. EHP was opened, as an outpatient facility, in June 1973. It was initially funded, for twenty-
nine months, by the federal government. 3 footnotes. 2
tables. 4 references.

7.190   Schramm, Carl J. "Measuring the Return on Program
Costs: Evaluation of a Multi-Employer Alcoholism

Treatment Program." <u>American Journal of Public Health</u>
67 (1977):   50-51.

The Johns Hopkins University School of Hygiene and Public Health, and the U.S. Department of Labor's Office
of Research and Development, established in Baltimore
in 1972 an alcoholism referral and treatment program
to serve multiple employers and unions. The program
was known as the Employee Health Program (EHP). This
study found this type of program to be a cost-effective
method of treatment for alcoholic workers. Author biographical information. 2 tables.

7.191   Schramm, Carl J., Wallace Mandell and Janet Archer.
<u>Workers Who Drink: Their Treatment in an Industrial
Setting</u>. Lexington, MA: D.C. Heath and Co., 1978.

This book is the result of a cooperative effort by researchers from Johns Hopkins University, private and
government employers, alcoholic employees, and unions
in the Baltimore, Maryland area.   38 tables.   3 figures.
15 notes.   73 references.

7.192   Schurtman, Robert. "The Effect of Psychodynamic Acti-
vation of Symbiotic Gratification Fantasies on Involvement in a Treatment Program for Alcoholics." <u>Disserta-
tion Abstracts International</u> 39:   6142B.   Ph.D. dissertation, New York University, 1978.   Order No. DA7912322.

Seventy-two inpatient alcoholics were divided into two
matched groups of thirty-six subjects each. All subjects
received subliminal stimulation. One group received an
experimental message. The other group received a neu-
tral control message. The group that received the experimental message became more involved in the alcoholism
treatment program than did the other group.

7.193   Seddon, John T., Jr. "Why Council Industrial Alcoholism
Programs Fail." <u>Labor-Management Alcoholism Journal</u> 7
(January-February 1978):   42-43.

Three administrative approaches responsible for the
failure of National Council on Alcoholism (NCA) industrial alcoholism programs. Author biographical information.

7.194   See, Jasper G. Chen. "Raising Funds for NCA: A Frus-
trating Job." <u>Labor-Management Alcoholism Journal</u> 9
(September-October 1979):   63-65.

Compares statistics regarding the number of cases of alcoholism and other diseases in the U.S. and how much
money is raised to combat these diseases. The stigma
associated with alcoholism is given as the main reason
it is difficult to raise money for alcoholism research

and treatment. The success of Alcoholics Anonymous
(AA)--an organization which refuses to accept financial assistance from individuals who do not belong to
AA--is lauded as the most successful in helping alcoholics. Author biographical information.

7.195   Senay, Edward C. "Alcohol." Chapter in <u>Substance Abuse</u>
<u>Disorders in Clinical Practice</u>, by Edward C. Senay, 31-
59. Littleton, MA: PSG Publishing Co., Inc., 1983.

Alcohol abuse and its treatment, including medical problems associated with alcohol abuse. Alcoholic coma, alcohol amblyopia, alcohol myopathy, liver disease, alcoholic hepatitis, pancreatitis, and gastritis are some
of these problems. 33 references.

7.196   Shain, Martin. "An Exploration of the Ability of Broad-
Based EAPS to Generate Alcohol-Related Referrals."
Chapter in <u>The Human Resources Management Handbook</u>:
<u>Principles and Practice of Employee Assistance Programs</u>,
edited by Samuel H. Klarreich, James L. Francek and C.
Eugene Moore, 232-242. New York, NY: Praeger Publish-
ers, 1985.

From the viewpoint of this study, broad-based programs
identified alcohol-related problems as well as did nar-
rower programs. 1 table. 18 references.

7.197   Shields, Michael. "Relaxation Therapy and Its Use in
the Treatment of Alcoholism." in <u>Counter Measures for</u>
<u>Alcoholism and Drug Abuse</u>, edited by Thomas M. Nelson
and Birendra K. Sinha, 233-238. Edmonton: University
of Alberta Department of Psychology and the Alberta Alcoholism and Drug Abuse Commission, 1972.

Autogenic training is used with alcoholics at the Alberta Alcoholism and Drug Abuse Commission (AADAC) in Edmonton, Alberta. Autogenic training is a method of relaxation therapy. This is a psycho-physiologic approach to tension reduction and involves mental and
bodily functions simultaneously. 4 references.

7.198   Shulman, Gerald D. "What Industry and Treatment Resources Need from Each Other." <u>Labor-Management Alco-</u>
<u>holism Journal</u> 8 (July-August 1978): 3-11.

A dual presentation--one by Gerald D. Shulman and the
other by Donald W. Magruder--about industrial alcoholism
programs and alcoholism treatment centers. Author biographical information. 2 photographs.

7.199   Silber, Austin. "The Contribution of Psychoanalysis to
the Treatment of Alcoholism." Chapter in <u>Alcoholism and</u>
<u>Clinical Psychiatry</u>, edited by Joel Solomon, 195-211.
New York, NY: Plenum Publishing Corp., 1982.

A clinical professor of psychiatry, from the New York
University Medical Center Psychoanalytic Institute,
talks about the contribution of psychoanalysis to the
treatment of alcoholism. The speaker bases his comments on his twenty years' experience with alcoholic
patients. 33 references.

7.200   Sladen, Bernard J. and Gerald J. Mozdzierz. "An MMPI
        Scale to Predict Premature Termination from Inpatient
        Alcohol Treatment." Journal of Clinical Psychology
        41 (November 1985): 855-862.

        A Minnesota Multiphasic Personality Inventory (MMPI)
        scale was used to differentiate completers from drop-
        outs in a four-week alcohol treatment program. The
        subjects were male veterans at the Hines Veterans Ad-
        ministration Hospital in Hines, Illinois. Twenty-one
        items were used to differentiate completers from drop-
        outs. Author biographical information. Abstract. 2
        tables. 2 footnotes. 22 references.

7.201   Small, Edward J., Jr. and Barry Leach. "Counseling
        Homosexual Alcoholics: Ten Case Histories." Journal
        of Studies on Alcohol 38 (1977): 2077-2086.

        Psychoanalytic viewpoints are related to homosexuality
        and alcoholism. None of the ten homosexuals fit the
        stereotype of the male homosexual. Author biographi-
        cal information. Abstract. 4 footnotes. 27 refer-
        ences.

7.202   Smart, Reginald G. "Employed Alcoholics Treated Vol-
        untarily and under Constructive Coercion: A Follow-Up
        Study." Quarterly Journal of Studies on Alcohol 35
        (1974):

        Compares employed alcoholics in Toronto, Ontario who
        were treated voluntarily to employed alcoholics who
        were treated under constructive coercion. The volun-
        tary patients showed more improvement than did the
        mandatory patients. The patients were from the May
        Street alcoholism unit and the Donwood Institute. Ab-
        stract. Author biographical information. 1 table. 12
        references.

7.203   Smart, Reginald G. and Gaye Gray. "Minimal, Moderate
        and Long-Term Treatment for Alcoholism." British Jour-
        nal of Addiction 73 (1978): 35-38.

        Data about alcoholics treated at twelve clinics in On-
        tario, Canada was used in this study. Major variables
        examined included the Alcoholic Involvement Scale, phys-
        ical health, motivation for treatment, social stability,
        and attitudes to abstinence. When alcoholics are matched
        for these variables, the variables support the value of

long-term treatment in promoting abstinence. Author
biographical information. 2 tables. 5 references.

7.204   Smith, Christopher J. "Locating Alcoholism Treatment
         Facilities." Economic Geography 59 (October 1983):
         368-385.

         Topics discussed include: alcoholism treatment facili-
         ties, the components of comprehensive service delivery,
         Pennsylvania as a case study, alcohol service delivery
         in Oklahoma, and explaining the locational pattern of
         alcohol treatment programs. Author biographical infor-
         mation. Abstract. 6 figures. 2 tables. 29 refer-
         ences.

7.205   Smithers, Francis C. "Why Don't We Stick with Success?"
         Labor-Management Alcoholism Journal 9 (July-August 1979):
         22-23.

         States why self-referral for alcoholism treatment is not
         an effective means of referral. Points out why referral
         should be based on poor job performance. Author bio-
         graphical information.

7.206   Sobell, Mark B. and Linda C. Sobell. "Alcoholics Treat-
         ed by Individualized Behavior Therapy: One Year Treat-
         ment Outcome." Behaviour Research and Therapy 11 (1973):
         599-618.

         Seventy male alcoholics, hospitalized at Patton State
         Hospital, volunteered to take part in this research.
         The authors concluded that some alcoholics, one year af-
         ter treatment, can maintain controlled drinking. An
         earlier version of this paper was presented at the Eight-
         ieth Annual Meeting, American Psychological Association,
         Honolulu, Hawaii, 1972. Author biographical information.
         Abstract. 3 figures. 4 tables. 17 references.

7.207   Soterakis, Jack and Frank L. Iber. "Increased Rate of
         Alcohol Removal from Blood with Oral Fructose and Su-
         crose." American Journal of Clincial Nutrition 28
         (March 1975): 254-257.

         Eight male, abstinent alcoholic patients took part in
         this study. Fructose and sucrose, compared to glucose,
         increased the rate of removal of alcohol from the blood
         of these volunteers. Alcohol was administered intrave-
         nously. Author biographical information. Abstract. 4
         figures. 19 references.

7.208   Southmayd, Edna B. "The Role of the Dietitian in Team
         Therapy for Chronic Alcoholism." Journal of the Ameri-
         can Dietetic Association 64 (February 1974): 184-186.

         Breakfast, between-meal eating, protein-fat-carbohydrates

and vitamins and minerals are discussed in relation to treating chronic alcoholism nutritionally. Author biographical information. 5 references.

7.209   Starr, David Rood. "A Study of the Occurrence and Characteristics of Burnout among Alcoholism-Treatment Professionals." Dissertation Abstracts International 41: 3430A. Ph.D. dissertation, University of Idaho, 1980. Order No. DA8100393,

The research sample for this study consisted of 203 alcoholism treatment professionals. They were members of the Alcoholism Professional Staff Society of Washington State. All were administered the Maslach Burnout Inventory and Tolor-Tamerin Attitudes toward Alcoholism Inventory. The sample consisted of men and women.

7.210   Steinglass, Peter. "Experimenting with Family Treatment Approaches to Alcoholism, 1950-1975: A Review." Family Process 15 (March 1976): 97-123.

Four main parts make up this article: the alcoholic marriage, concurrent group therapy for alcoholics and spouses, the adaptation of family theory to alcoholism therapy, and family therapy techniques. Abstract. Author biographical information. 46 references.

7.211   Stern, Barbara F. "The Effect of an Explicit Treatment Contract in an Alcohol Inpatient Setting." Dissertation Abstracts International 35: 1928B. Ph.D. dissertation, Boston College, 1974. Order No. DA7421819.

Forty male and female subjects between the ages of twenty-five and sixty participated in this study. The subjects had been voluntarily admitted to an inpatient alcohol treatment center. The subjects were assigned to one of four contract groups. Three hypotheses were tested.

7.212   Stolt, G. "Rehabilitation of the Alcoholic in Sweden." British Journal of Addiction Supplement No. 1, 70 (April 1975): 35-41.

Five people discuss rehabilitation of the alcoholic in Sweden. Author biographical information. 1 figure. 1 reference.

7.213   Sugerman, A. Arthur. "Alcoholism: An Overview of Treatment Models and Methods." Chapter in Alcohol, Science and Society Revisited, edited by Edith Lisansky Gomberg, Helene Raskin White and John A. Carpenter, 262-278. Ann Arbor, MI: University of Michigan Press, 1982.

Six treatment models are examined: the medical model, the behavior modification model, the psychological model,

the social model, the Alcoholics Anonymous (AA) model
and the multivariant model. Also dealt with in this
chapter: acute alcoholic states, outpatient and inpatient detoxification, and the post-withdrawal phase.
11 references.

7.214   Swint, J. Michael and William B. Nelson. "The Appli-
        cation of Economic Analysis to Evaluation of Alcoholism
        Rehabilitation Programs." Inquiry 14 (March 1977):
        63-72.

        The application of economic analysis to the evaluation
        of alcoholism rehabilitation programs is examined with
        the aid of cost-benefit analysis (CBA), and the develop-
        ment of an algorithm and case study. Author biographi-
        cal information. 5 tables. 26 references and notes.

7.215   Swint, J. Michael, Michael Decker and David R. Lairson.
        "The Economic Returns to Employment-Based Alcoholism Pro-
        grams: A Methodology." Journal of Studies on Alcohol
        39 (1978): 1633-1639.

        The economic model presented can be used to evaluate
        profit-oriented alcoholism rehabilitation programs. The
        model can be used to analyze all future economic savings
        of the organization that utilizes the model. This eco-
        nomic model can also examine retrospective costs of re-
        habilitating alcoholic employees. Author biographical
        information. Abstract. 6 footnotes. 20 references.

7.216   Swinyard, Chester A., Shakuntala Chaube and David B.
        Sutton. "Neurological and Behavioral Aspects of Tran-
        scendental Meditation Relevant to Alcoholism: A Review."
        Annals of the New York Academy of Sciences 233 (1974):
        162-173.

        Transcendental meditation (TM) may be helpful in prevent-
        ing alcoholism by raising an individual's tolerance to
        stress, thereby curtailing a need for alcohol. TM may
        also be of value to alcoholics who have achieved sobriety
        by helping them adjust to life without alcohol. Author
        biographical information. 12 figures. 37 references.

7.217   Taylor, John R., John E. Helzer and Lee N. Robins.
        "Moderate Drinking in Ex-Alcoholics: Recent Studies."
        Journal of Studies on Alcohol 47 (1986): 115-121.

        Reviews literature published since 1976 on moderate
        drinking in ex-alcoholics. Strict comparisons of studies
        is difficult for various reasons, including definitions
        of moderate drinking. Abstinence--not moderate drink-
        ing--would appear to be the realistic treatment goal for
        most alcoholics. Author biographical information. Ab-
        stract. 25 references.

7.218   Taylor, Mary Catherine. "Alcoholics Anonymous: How It
        Works Recovery Processes in a Self-Help Group." Disser-
        tation Abstracts International 39: 7532A. Ph.D. dis-
        sertation, University of California, San Francisco,
        1977. Order No. DA7913241.

        Investigates the recovery process for alcoholics in Al-
        coholics Anonymous (AA). Distinct stages of recovery
        are identified.

7.219   Topolnicki, Denise M. "Where to Take a Drug or Drinking
        Problem." Money 15 (January 1986): 120-122, 124 and
        126-128.

        The Smithers Alcoholism Treatment and Training Center,
        Alcoholics Anonymous (AA), Betty Ford Center, and the
        Schick Shadel Hospital are among the many places to re-
        ceive help for alcoholism. 7 photographs.

7.220   Tozzi, Susan Mary. "The Effects of Levels of Self-Es-
        teem and Self-Motivation on Improvement During Treat-
        ment in Alcoholics." Dissertation Abstracts Interna-
        tional 46: 2827B. Ph.D. dissertation, Fordham Univer-
        sity, 1985. Order No. DA8521420.

        White male alcoholics, who were admitted to a thirty-day
        alcohol treatment program, were administered the Minne-
        sota Multiphasic Personality Inventory (MMPI), and the
        Rosenberg Self-Esteem Scale (RSE) as part of the author's
        research.

7.221   Trice, Harrison M. "Evaluation of Consultants and Coor-
        dinators." Labor-Management Alcoholism Journal 7 (No-
        vember-December 1977): 29-34.

        Reports on two studies: "Evaluation of the Occupational
        Program Consultant System for Alcoholism in New York
        State" and "Evaluation of Performance by Alcoholism Pro-
        gram Coordinators in the Northeast." Author biographi-
        cal information. 1 photograph.

7.222   Trice, Harrison M. and Janice M. Beyer. "Social Control
        in Worksettings: Using the Constructive Confrontation
        Strategy with Problem-Drinking Employees." Journal of
        Drug Issues 12 (1982): 21-49.

        Main topics covered include: the background of the con-
        cept of social control; social controls and deviant be-
        havior; social controls of problem drinking in work set-
        tings--the strategy of constructive confrontation; bases
        of the strategy; history of the strategy; competition
        and cooptation; evidence of success; problems with im-
        plementation of the strategy; unintended consequences;
        and changes in the workforce. Author biographical in-
        formation. Abstract. 4 notes. 160 references.

7.223   Trice, Harrison M. and Paul M. Roman. "Treatment of the
        Deviant Drinker: Alcoholics Anonymous." in Spirits and
        Demons at Work: Alcohol and Other Drugs on the Job, by
        Harrison M. Trice and Paul M. Roman, Second Edition,
        213-225. Ithaca, NY: New York State School of Industri-
        al and Labor Relations Cornell University, 1978.

        Describes the success of Alcoholics Anonymous (AA) in
        the treatment of deviant drinkers. Also talks about the
        limitations of AA with certain alcoholics.

7.224   Trice, Harrison M. and Paul M. Roman. "Treatment of the
        Deviant Drinker: Other Strategies." in Spirits and
        Demons at Work: Alcohol and Other Drugs on the Job, by
        Harrison M. Trice and Paul M. Roman, Second Edition, 225-
        227. Ithaca, NY: New York State School of Industrial
        and Labor Relations Cornell University, 1978.

        Drug therapy, conditioned reflex therapy, and group
        therapies are options to Alcoholics Anonymous (AA) in
        the treatment of the deviant drinker.

7.225   Trotter, Robert J. "The Antabuse High." Science News
        118 (September 13, 1980): 173.

        Research by Zavie W. Brown and Zalman Amit of Concordia
        University in Montreal. Brown and Amit did an experi-
        ment with two drugs used in alcoholism treatment pro-
        grams. The researchers discovered that those partici-
        pants in the experiment who had taken the drugs antabuse
        and temposil became more intoxicated than the subjects
        who had taken a placebo.

7.226   Turner, David Francis. "The Rey Method of Memory Re-
        training: Its Validity, and Usefulness as an Aid to the
        Psychotherapeutic Treatment of Alcoholism." Disserta-
        tion Abstracts International 47: 808B. Ph.D. disserta-
        tion, University of Houston, 1985. Order No. DA8607040.

        Thirty long-term male alcoholics, being treated in a
        four-week inpatient psychotherapeutic program, were the
        subjects in this study. The subjects were assigned to
        three experimental groups. The Rey Method was found to
        significantly improve the memory of the experimental
        group which took part in memory retraining.

7.227   Vail, Shirley Smith. "The Recovering Alcoholic: Dura-
        tion of Abstinence and Personality Change." Disserta-
        tion Abstracts International 35: 3601B-3602B. Ph.D.
        dissertation, Wayne State University, 1974. Order No.
        DA7429876.

        The sample for this research, which tested two hypothe-
        ses, were men and women in Oakland County, Michigan.
        The sample included seventy-four members of six

Alcoholics Anonymous (AA) groups and a comparison group of twenty-two nonalcoholic peers.

7.228   Vaillant, George E., William Clark, Catherine Cyrus, Eva S. Milofsky, Jeffrey Kopp, Victoria Wells Wulsin and Nancy P. Mogielnicki. "Prospective Study of Alcoholism Treatment: Eight-Year Follow-Up." American Journal of Medicine 75 (September 1983): 455-463.

The subjects for this study were inpatients at the Cambridge and Somerville Program for Alcohol Rehabilitation at the Cambridge, Massachusetts Hospital. Eight years after treatment, 29% of the patients had died, 26% continued to have serious alcohol problems, and 25% had achieved abstinence. The patients were one hundred men and women. The Straus-Bacon Scale is a major research tool used in this investigation. Author biographical information. Abstract. 1 figure. 4 tables. 50 references.

7.229   Van Wagner, Richard W. "A Simple Measure of Program Effectiveness." Labor-Management Alcoholism Journal 8 (September-October 1978): 62-63.

Information required to determine the effectiveness of an employee alcoholism program (EAP). Author biographical information. 1 photograph.

7.230   Viamontes, Jorge A. "Review of Drug Effectiveness in the Treatment of Alcoholism." American Journal of Psychiatry 128 (June 1972): 1570-1571.

British and American literature--eighty-nine studies-- was reviewed by the author. He questions the claims made in the papers, particularly the methodologies used. Paraldehyde, hydroxyzine, metronidazole, and meprobamate are four of the drugs discussed in the papers. Abstract. Author biographical information. 2 tables. 7 references.

7.231   Visocan, Barbara J. "Nutritional Management of Alcoholism." Journal of the American Dietetic Association 83 (December 1983): 693-696.

Focuses on the nutritional hazards of alcoholism, the team approach to alcoholism, and the role of the dietician in alcohol rehabilitation. Assessment, planning, implementation, and evaluation constitute the dietician's course of action. Author biographical information. 2 tables. 31 references.

7.232   "Vocational Recovery: NCA's Employment Program for Recovered Alcoholics." Labor-Management Alcoholism Journal 10 (May-June 1981): 243-245.

The National Council on Alcoholism (NCA) began its Employment Program for Recovered Alcoholics (EPRA) on
January 1, 1977. Union Carbide, in the mid-1970s,
provided the NCA with assistance in the establishment
of the program. The program is currently funded by
the New York City Department of Education, the New York
State Bureau of Alcoholism Services, and the New York
State Office of Vocational Rehabilitation.

7.233 Walsh, Diana Chapman. "Employee Assistance Programs."
       Milbank Memorial Fund Quarterly 60 (Summer 1982): 492-
       517.

       The first part of this article consists of a definition
       and history of employee assistance. This is followed by
       a discussion of the limitations of the job-performance
       criterion as the major reason for referring an employee
       for help. Problems other than alcoholism are being ac-
       cepted as valid grounds for assisting employees. The
       pros and cons of in-house programs versus outside con-
       tracting are also covered, as is the issue of cost-ef-
       fectiveness. Author biographical information. 2 fig-
       ures. 39 references.

7.234 Ware, Claude Thomas. "Relationship of Pre-Treatment and
       Treatment Variables to Sobriety in Alcoholics Ninety
       Days after Therapy." Dissertation Abstracts Interna-
       tional 35: 1445B. Ph.D. dissertation, United States
       International University, 1974. Order No. DA7420553.

       Twenty-one alcoholism counselors provided data about
       215 alcoholics, who were the subjects for this investi-
       gation in which three hypotheses were tested.

7.235 Waring, Mary L. and Inez Sperr. "A Comparative Study
       of Male and Female Bartenders: Their Potential for As-
       sisting in the Prevention of Alcohol Abuse." Journal
       of Alcohol and Drug Education 28 (Fall 1982): 1-11.

       Sixty-four bartenders--twenty female and forty-four
       male--were interviewed by the authors. The bartenders
       were employed in forty-three bars in a southern U.S.
       community. The behavior of the bartenders toward their
       customers and the bartenders' drinking patterns were
       two areas investigated by the authors. Author biograph-
       ical information. Abstract. 4 tables. 20 references.

7.236 Wasserstein, Joyce R. "Alcoholic Patients' Perceptions
       of Nonalcoholic and Recovering Alcoholic Counselors Dur-
       ing Treatment." Dissertation Abstracts International
       46: 318B. Ph.D. dissertation, Ohio State University,
       1984. Order No. DA8504095.

       The Counselor Rating Form, Tennessee Self-Concept Scale,

Counselor Behavior Scale, and Treatment Evaluation Form
were used in this research. The subjects were sixty
Black, male alcoholics.

7.237 Westermeyer, Joseph. "Treatment of Alcohol Abuse: Psychotherapies and Sociotherapies." Chapter in Treatment
Aspects of Drug Dependence, edited by Arnold Schecter,
223-234. West Palm Beach, FL: CRC Press, Inc., 1978.

Psychotherapies: relaxation methods, behavior modification, family therapy, group therapy, marathon group
therapy, psychodrama, transactional analysis, and crisis
theory. Sociotherapies: contingency management, education and training, occupational and industrial programs.
Self-help programs and religiotherapies: Alcoholics
Anonymous (AA), Alanon, Alateen, Salvation Army, religious conversion, and high-risk group activities. Social planning of treatment systems: systems planning,
acute care facilities, hospitalization, partial hospitalization, residential facilities, and outpatient care.
34 references.

7.238 "Where VIP's Go to Conquer the Bottle." U.S. News and
World Report 86 (March 19, 1979): 8.

Alcoholism treatment has been available at the Long
Beach Naval Hospital since 1970. The hospital claims
a 75% treatment success rate. People with celebrity
and non-celebrity status undergo rehabilitation.

7.239 Whitehead, Paul C. "The Prevention of Alcoholism: Di-
vergences and Convergences of Two Approaches." Addictive Diseases 1 (1975): 431-443.

Two models--the sociocultural model and the distribution
of consumption model--are discussed in relation to the
prevention of alcoholism. Author biographical information. 10 notes. 44 references.

7.240 Whitfield, Charles L., Goff Thompson, Anita Lamb, Vivian
Spencer, Michael Pfeifer and Mary Browning-Ferrando.
"Detoxification of 1,024 Alcoholic Patients without Psychoactive Drugs." Journal of the American Medical Association 239 (April 3, 1978): 1409-1410.

College graduates were successful in providing reassur-
ance and reality orientation to alcoholic patients, who
underwent detoxification quickly, safely, and without
the use of psychoactive drugs. Author biographical information. Abstract. 2 tables. 12 references.

7.241 Williams, Florence. "Psychological, Demographic, and
Supportive System Variables Associated with Recovery of
Hospitalized Alcoholics." Dissertation Abstracts Inter-
national 46: 668B. Ph.D. dissertation, United States

International University, 1978. Order No. DA8508428.

Sixty alcoholics--male and female--took part in this research. They were part of a in-hospital alcoholism rehabilitation program. Self-esteem, drinking attitude,
and anxiety were three psychological variables measured.
Milieu therapy was one important aspect of the treatment program.

7.242   Williams, Richard L. and Joseph Tramontana. "The Eval-
        uation of Occupational Alcoholism Programs." Chapter in
        Alcoholism and Its Treatment in Industry, edited by Carl
        J. Schramm, 109-135. Baltimore, MD: Johns Hopkins Uni-
        versity Press, 1977.

        Deals with factors limiting the adequacy of program
        evaluations, presents a model for evaluating occupation-
        al alcoholism programs (OAPs), discusses designs for
        evaluating the effectiveness of these programs, talks
        about frequency rates for evaluating program effective-
        ness, and concludes with the application of an evalua-
        tion model. 2 footnotes. 1 table. 25 references.

7.243   Willoughby, Alan. "Alcoholics Anonymous." Chapter in
        The Alcohol Troubled Person: Known and Unknown, by Alan
        Willoughby, 171-179. Chicago, IL: Nelson-Hall, Inc.,
        1979.

        A look at how both Alcoholics Anonymous (AA) and profes-
        sionals deal with the alcoholic person.

7.244   Wilson, Arthur S., Edward A. Mabry and Khalil A. Khavari.
        "Use of MMPI Profiles for Occupational Classification of
        Alcoholics." Journal of Studies on Alcohol 38 (1977):
        471-476.

        Nearly 1000 male alcoholics constituted the sample for
        this research. Minnesota Multiphasic Personality Inven-
        tory (MMPI) profile scores for these individuals were
        analyzed. Subjects from blue-collar occupations repre-
        sented the most accurate classification of alcoholics.
        The men were first treated for alcoholism between 1966
        and 1974. Abstract. Author biographical information.
        3 tables. 13 references.

7.245   Wilson, G. Terence, Russell C. Leaf and Peter E. Nathan.
        "The Aversive Control of Excessive Alcohol Consumption
        by Chronic Alcoholics in the Laboratory Setting." Jour-
        nal of Applied Behavior Analysis 8 (Spring 1975): 13-
        26.

        The research setting for three experiments was the Alco-
        hol Behavior Research Laboratory (ABRL) at Rutgers Uni-
        versity. The subjects were male alcoholics who had been
        treated unsuccessfully in various institutions in New

Jersey and New York State. Fourteen subjects took part
in the three experiments. Author biographical information. Abstract. 3 figures. 1 table. 23 references.

7.246   Zimberg, Sheldon. "Office Psychotherapy of Alcoholism."
Chapter in <u>Alcoholism and Clinical Psychiatry</u>, edited by
Joel Solomon, 213-229. New York, NY: Plenum Publishing
Corp., 1982.

This psychiatrist contends that, contrary to the experience of most psychiatrists, alcoholism is treatable in a
psychiatric office setting. To support his claim, he
cites statistics from a study of twenty-three alcoholics.
He also presents his findings in table form. 1 figure.
4 tables. 19 references.

Author Index

Numbers Refer to Entries, Not to Pages

Subject Index

Rodriguez, Joseph, 2.029
Roethke, Theodore, 5.099
role; confusion, 6.010; dif-
 ferences, 6.020; modeling,
 1.030
Room, R., 1.067
Roosevelt Hospital (New York
 City), 5.011
Rosenberg Self-Esteem Scale
 (RSE), 6.011, 7.220
Royal College of Psychia-
 trists (Britain), 1.002,
 5.118
Royal Columbian Hospital (New
 Westminster, B.C.), 5.060
Royal Edinburgh Hospital
 (Scotland), 1.024
Royal National Mission to
 Deep Sea Fishermen, 5.114
Rush, Benjamin, 1.007
Russia, see Soviet Union
Rutgers Center of Alcohol
 Studies, 1.008, 2.204
Rutgers University Alcohol
 Behavior Research Laborato-
 ry (ABRL), 7.245
Ryder, Donald, 3.043

Sadler, Marion, 3.024
safety, see accidents
Salford Health Authority
 (Britain), 1.027
Salvation Army, 7.237; Canada, 7.147; Auckland, New
 Zealand, 1.165
Saskatchewan, 5.060, 5.076
schizophrenia, 7.152
Schofield/Colgan, 7.005
Scotland, 1.023, 1.033, 1.055,
 5.001, 5.030, 5.114, 6.001,
 6.067
seamen, 5.105, 5.106, 5.114
seconal, 7.077
secretaries, 7.175
Seixas, Frank A., 5.015
Self-Administered Alcoholism
 Screening Test (SAAST),
 1.097
self-concept, see self-esteem
self-confidence, 7.085
Self-Disclosure Scale, 6.043
self-esteem, 1.152, 6.010,
 6.018, 6.036, 6.056, 6.063,
 6.078, 7.055, 7.121, 7.220,

7.241
self-image, see self-esteem
self-motivation, 7.220
seminars, see conferences
senators (U.S.), 4.026, 4.029,
 4.062
serax, 7.077
Serebro, Boris, 7.091
serum acetate level, 1.097
serum alcohol levels, 7.141
Serum Glutamic Oxaloacetic
 Transaminase (SGOT), 1.033
Services for Traffic Safety
 Project (Boston, Massachusetts), 7.009
Session Satisfaction Questionnaire, 7.128
Seven Oaks General Hospital
 (Winnipeg, Manitoba), 5.060
Severity of Alcohol Dependence
 Questionnaire (SADQ), 1.031,
 1.033, 1.145
sex roles, 6.010, 6.038, 6.056,
 6.065, 6.078, 6.080
sexism, 6.058
sexuality, 6.006, 6.010, 6.025,
 6.026, 6.031
shame, 1.155
Shaw, Stan, 1.067
Sherman, Paul A., 5.015
Short Alcohol Dependence Data
 (SADD)(questionnaire), 1.033
Short Michigan Alcoholism Screening Test, 1.048
Shulman, Gerald D., 7.198
sick leave, 2.091, 3.010, 7.104
Siksay, Nick, 2.126
Silbermann, Eugene, 3.064
SimuFlite Lear 55 simulator,
 5.024, 5.059, 5.083
Sixteen Personality Factor Questionnaire, 4.036
Sixteen Personality Factor Questionnaire (16PF), Form A,
 7.135
skid row, 2.128, 3.010
skin musculoskeletal system,
 1.103, 1.143
small businesses, 2.062, 2.118
Smith, Alfred A., 2.234
sobriety, 3.017, 5.096, 6.028,
 7.129, 7.148, 7.172, 7.216
social class, 5.018, 6.071
social integration, 1.073

Company Name Index

Directory of Sources

For more information about University Microfilms International (UMI) dissertations, and National Technical Information Service (NTIS) publications, write to:

University Microfilms International
300 North Zeeb Road
Ann Arbor, Michigan
48106

National Technical Information Service
5285 Port Royal Road
Springfield, Virginia
22161

About the Compiler

JOHN J. MILETICH is Reference Librarian at the University of Alberta, Canada. He has compiled a number of major bibliographies, including *Retirement: An Annotated Bibliography* (Greenwood Press, 1986).